Münzenberg

The Orthopedic Shoe

Indications and Prescription

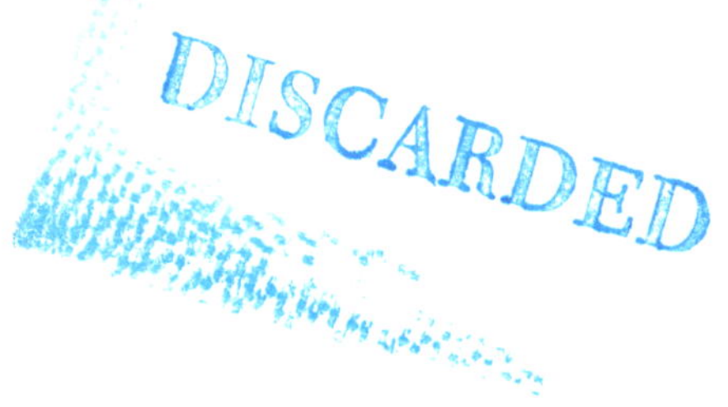

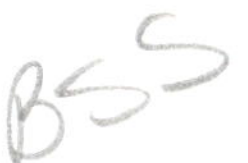

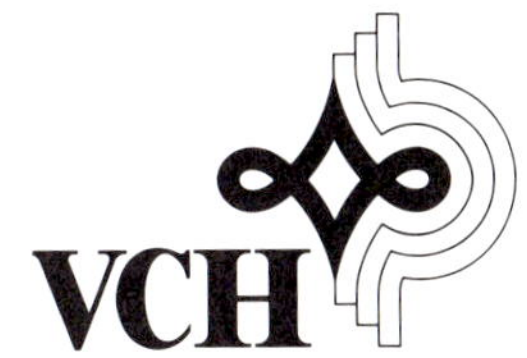

© VCH Verlagsgesellschaft mbH, D-6940 Weinheim (Federal Republic of Germany), 1985

Distribution:

VCH Verlagsgesellschaft, P.O. Box 1260/1280, D-6940 Weinheim (Federal Republic of Germany)

USA and Canada: VCH Publishers, 303 N.W. 12th Avenue, Deerfield Beach, FL 33442-1705 (USA)

ISBN 3-527-15227-X (VCH Verlagsgesellschaft)
ISBN 0-89573-429-X (VCH Publishers)

The Orthopedic Shoe

Indications and Prescription

by K. Joachim Münzenberg

translated by
David Beattie

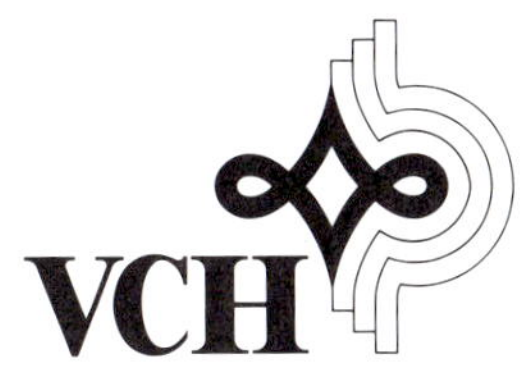

Original title: Der orthopädische Schuh – Indikation und Rezeptur
By K. Joachim Münzenberg
Published by VCH Verlagsgesellschaft
Copyright © VCH Verlagsgesellschaft mbH, D-6940 Weinheim, 1983

Prof. Dr. med. K. Joachim Münzenberg
Orthopädische Universitätsklinik
Sigmund-Freud-Str. 25
D-5300 Bonn-Venusberg
Federal Republic of Germany

The authors and publisher have made every effort to ensure that drug selection and dosage described in this book are in accord with current recommendations and practice at the time of publication. However, in view of changes in regulations and ongoing research with regard to drug actions and therapeutic schemes – but also in view of potential typographical errors – neither the authors nor the publisher are to be held responsible for the accuracy of the statements made. Rather, the reader is urged to study the package insert for indications, dosage, warnings and precautions before administering a drug. This is particularly important when the drug under considerations is new or infrequently used.

Translator: David Beattie
Illustrator: Lothar Knorn
Editorial Director: Silvia Osteen
Production Director: Maximilian Montkowski
Production Manager: Peter J. Biel

Deutsche Bibliothek Cataloguing-in-Publication Data

Münzenberg, K. Joachim:
The orthopedic shoe: indications and prescription / by K. Joachim Münzenberg. Transl. by David Beattie. [Ill.: Lothar Knorn]. – Weinheim; Deerfield Beach, FL: VCH, 1985.
   Dt. Ausg. u. d. T.: Münzenberg, K. Joachim: Der orthopädische Schuh
   ISBN 3-527-15227-X (Weinheim)
   ISBN 0-89573-429-X (Deerfield Beach)

Composition, Printing and Bookbinding: Zechnersche Buchdruckerei, D-6720 Speyer
Printed in the Federal Republic of Germany

To Marshall R. Urist

Foreword

We have to thank Germany for the preservation into the last quarter of the twentieth century of the almost lost art of the classical orthopedic shoemaker, the perfectionist who not only clads the crippled foot but so understands foot mechanics that his product can correct or prevent further deformity. In this book, sympathetically translated by David Beattie, English speakers can share this knowledge and enjoy the insights into disordered foot mechanisms. The text is set out logically and readably and the 64 black and white illustrations are clear and informative. This is a book, as the title makes clear, primarily for those orthopedic surgeons and orthotists who treat foot conditions where what one might call the "texture" of the foot is normal. Congenital deformities, amputations, alterations of foot shape due to surgery, accidents or paralyses, all these are classified and catalogued here with great care. Less emphasis has been placed on the foot problems of sufferers from arthritis in whom the "texture" and structure of the foot is abnormal and for whom the main consideration is to provide a lightweight "package" for a delicate object of variable geometry. But all those who come in contact with the medical (as opposed to the orthopedic surgical) problems of the foot will need to read this book, if only because there is such a dearth of expert orthotic advice that any physicians interested in foot problems will find such patients turning up in their clinics. Physicians as well as surgeons will want to read this book for the pleasure of "listening in" to the knowledge of the author who so obviously knows and loves his job and has an equal expertise in explaining it.

Bath, April 1985   A. St. J. Dixon

Preface

It would be no exaggeration at all to say that the orthopedic shoe has often occupied a somewhat neglected position in the therapeutic arsenal available to the medical profession. Similarly, books for ready reference in this field are particularly few and far between. It is hoped that this small volume will remedy that situation. I do not claim that it is complete, and readers are bound to draw my attention to certain aspects that have been omitted. For example, matters pertaining to materials are mentioned in exceptional cases only. However, excellent monographs on this particular subject already exist, and there is so little to choose between the wide range of present-day materials in terms of quality that it should in most cases be left to the shoemaker to decide on the preferred material in the light of personal experience.

My grateful thanks are due to L. Knorn who prepared the illustrations with great understanding and much skill. Anyone possessing more than passing familiarity with the specialist literature on the orthopedic shoe will know that standard illustrations occur in numerous publications. We did not see it as our duty to feign originality by re-working illustrations which have stood the test of time. I am particularly indebted here to the works of Regenspurger, Marquardt and Kraus.

My enthusiasm for the orthopedic shoe was first kindled by my friend and teacher, F. Henkel (Master Orthopedic Shoe Technician) in Göttingen. He generously allowed me to become intimately familiar with every aspect of his workshop and was a constant source of sound advice. My thanks are also due to M. Montkowski of VCH Publishers for his suggestions concerning the graphic layout of this volume, and to P. J. Biel for his acknowledged care in the typesetting. I owe a special debt of gratitude to Silvia Osteen for her critical perusal of the manuscript.

Bonn, April 1985   K. Joachim Münzenberg

Contents

1 The Shoe

Because it is of central importance in the manufacture of the shoe and because it also helps us to understand the function of certain orthopedic elements, the *shoe last* will be considered first. The last is a three-dimensional replica of the human foot and is made of wood or some other material over which the shoemaker constructs the shoe (Fig. 1). Like the foot, the last is also thought of as having a sole. Thus, if we imagine the last to be a foot, the sole of

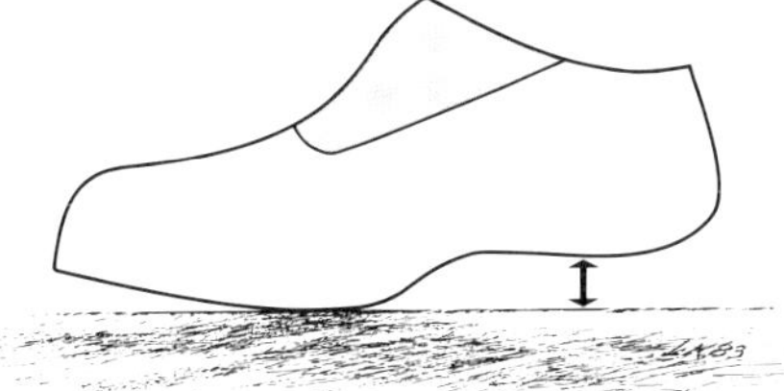

Fig. 1. Last for low shoe (↕ heel pitch)

the last is that part which would correspond to the sole of the foot. However, there is one difference: because the sole of the last faces upwards during shoe manufacture, the shoemaker speaks of the "top" when referring to the sole of the last, and the "bottom" when meaning the dorsal area of the last.

1.1 Parts of the Shoe

A shoe consists of the shoe bottom and the upper (Fig. 2). These two components may be attached in a wide variety of ways using adhesive or stitching techniques.

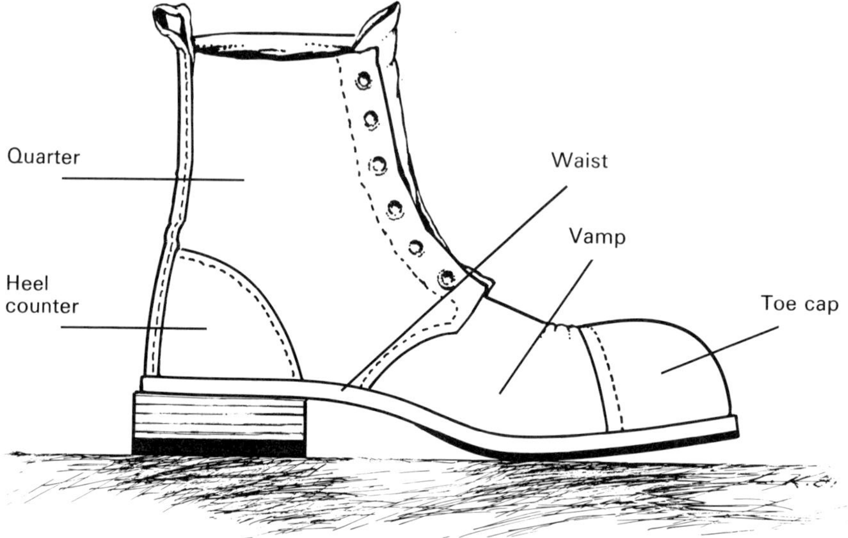

Fig. 2. Ankle boot (high shoe) with component parts illustrated (Derby upper)

1.1.1 Shoe Bottom

The *shoe bottom* comprises the insole and the outsole, the bottom filler, the waist and the heel.

1.1.1.1 Insole

To a certain extent the insole is the basic element which determines the shape of the shoe (see Fig. 20). The shoe is constructed over the insole and, at one time, the most weighty discussions over correct shoe shape concerned the various possible insole designs. This is still true today, although perhaps no longer in quite such a dogmatic and absolute way as in the past. In the case of a child's foot, for example, the insole should ensure that the smaller the foot (i.e. the younger the child), the more space there is for the forefoot.

During shoe construction the insole is first directly fitted and placed over the sole of the last, i.e. that part of the last which corresponds to the sole of the foot.

The uppers and the shoe bottom are then attached at the edge of the insole which thus becomes the connecting element between the uppers and the shoe bottom. The insole should be made of leather because this material possesses the best moisture-absorbing properties and is also relatively slip-resistant. An additional piece of thin material, the *whole-length sock,* may be glued on top of the insole.

1.1.1.2 Outsole

The outsole is that part of the shoe which comes into contact with the ground or floor. It may be constructed as a *full-length sole,* in which case it extends from the heel to the toe of the shoe, or as a *half-sole* which extends from the toe to the waist of the shoe and is placed over an additional full-length sole. Very robust shoes often also have a *midsole* sandwiched between the outsole and the insole; the midsole may be of varying length. In orthopedic shoe technology the midsole is an important element in the correction of leg inequality.

When the shoe is standing on a flat surface, the toe-end of the outsole is raised and is not in contact with the ground. This feature is referred to as the *toe spring,* and the angle of the toe spring depends on the height of the heel and the flexibility of the materials from which the shoe bottom and uppers are constructed. With low heels the toe spring should be slightly higher because, in such cases, the shoe bottom is under greater bending stress. The same applies when the shoe material is less flexible because rollover is facilitated by a slightly higher toe spring.

The outsole may be made of leather, rubber or a crêpe-like plastic material.

1.1.1.3 Bottom Filler

The bottom filler is the material placed in the cavity between the insole and (full-length) outsole. It compensates for unevenness in the forefoot area and its elastic properties cause pressure to be distributed over the entire sole of the foot (see Fig. 20). The bottom filler should not be too hard or too heavy and, for this reason, leather is generally not suitable. The material used must have good insulating properties and be capable of absorbing and giving off moisture. These requirements are best fulfilled by pressed or ground cork.

1.1.1.4 Waist

The waist is the underpart of the shoe from the heel seat to the joint, i.e. it is the part of the sole which is generally not in contact with the ground (see Fig. 2). Ideally, it should be elastic and slightly flexible around its longitudinal axis, but it should not be too elastic. In retail shoes (and in orthopedic shoes in certain indications), the waist of the shoe is generally reinforced with a metal plate (shank) which is inserted between the insole and the outsole and extends forward from the heel seat to the forepart of the foot.

The *waist of the last* refers to the height of the arch (or concavity) compared with the heel pitch and corresponds to the waist of the shoe (see Fig. 1). It must be consistent with the height of the heel. If the waist of the last (and therefore the heel) is too high, the toe spring will be reduced; this will produce transverse creasing of the upper over the joint line. If the waist of the last is too low, the tension of the upper leather over the toes will be reduced.

1.1.1.5 Heel

The heel is that part of the shoe which is attached to the sole underneath the seat of the shoe and is the first part to make contact with the ground during the strike phase of walking. Heel height has always been a vexed question in the many different schools of thought regarding correct footwear, and the shoe heel runs a close second to the variations in insole shape as the mainstay of sales in the fashion world. Nowadays, a height of 30 to 45 mm (1.2 to 1.8 inches) on ladies' shoes and 25 to 35 mm (1 to 1.4 inches) on men's shoes is considered normal.

The *seat lift* is the leather strip which is inserted between the convex seat region of the full-length sole and the heel in order to provide a level surface for the heel and to blend in with the sole.

The heel is intended to protect the foot from climatic conditions underfoot, and to improve and enhance walking performance. It increases the non-slip properties of the shoe, especially during downhill walking, and it relieves pressure on the longitudinal arch of the foot.

1.1.2 Upper

The *upper* consists of three main parts: the vamp and the two quarters.

1.1.2.1 Vamp

The vamp forms the forepart of the upper and it covers the forefoot. A toe cap may be placed over the toe-end of the vamp (Fig. 2).

1.1.2.2 Quarters

The two quarters cover the medial and lateral hindfoot and thus form the backpart of the outside of the upper. Generally, the medial and lateral quarters meet at the back of the shoe at the back seam; however, there are certain shoe designs in which one single quarter encases the entire heel of the foot.

The reinforcement of the quarters placed at the back of the shoe is known as the *heel counter*. The *lacing* is attached to the quarters of the shoe.

The small metal rings set in the leather facing stay of the quarter are the *eyelets,* and the *lace hooks* are the metal hooks which hold the lace for fastening.

The *tongue* of the shoe is situated beneath the lacing. In fact, it forms part of the vamp because it is either cut with it in one piece or stitched to it. If it is stitched to the quarters on both sides, it is known as a *bellows tongue.*

The *side linings* (see Fig. 20) are pieces of reinforcing material generally placed on each side of the shoe between the outside leather and the lining of the upper. They are thus positioned at the sides between the vamp and the quarters.

The height of the upper is measured in the line of the medial malleolus. A *shoe* (or *low shoe*) is one in which the quarters only rise to below the malleolus. An *ankle boot* (or *high shoe*) has an upper which is approximately 14 cm (5.6 inches) high. Boots in which the upper rises even higher are known as *half-boots* or *knee boots.*

The style of upper most commonly used in orthopedic shoes is the *Derby:* in this style the quarters are stitched on top of the vamp (see Fig. 2). Conversely, when the vamp overlays the quarters, the style is known as the *Oxford.* In the case of the *Balmoral,* the vamp continues in one piece along both sides of the shoe as far as the back seam, with the result that the quarters have to be stitched to the vamp rather than to the shoe bottom. A court shoe, for example, could be described as an incompletely developed Balmoral because it has no quarters.

1.2 Shoe Types

Individual shoe types are distinguished broadly in terms of the shape of the upper and the height of the heel. The upper is described as being open if the vamp or quarters are interrupted or totally absent, with the result that the

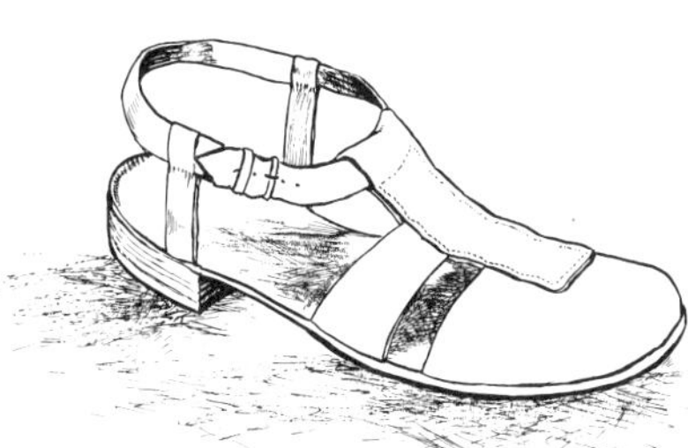

Fig. 3. Sandal

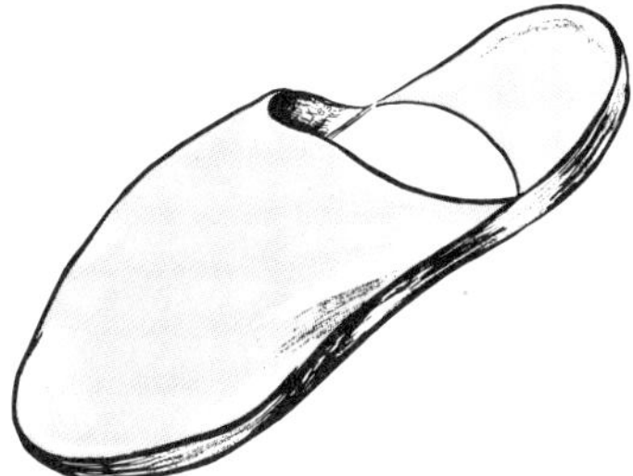

Fig. 4. Slipper

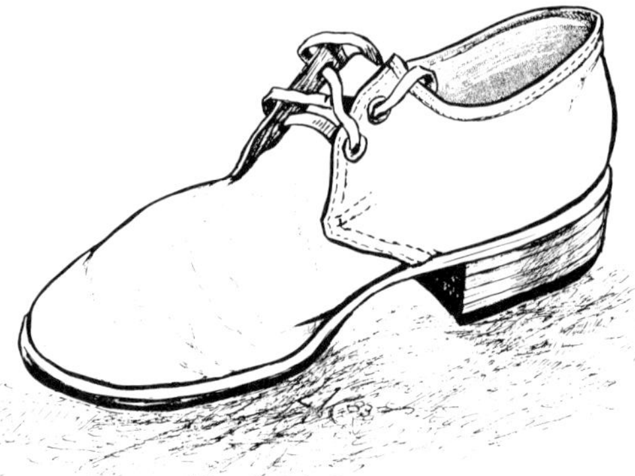

Fig. 5. Low shoe

upper does not rise continuously from the entire rim of the shoe bottom. Shoe types with open uppers include *sandals* and *slippers* (Fig. 3 and Fig. 4).

In the sandal, a strap (a remnant of the quarters) passes around the heel of the foot, and the vamp is not continuous.

In the slipper the upper consists simply of a vamp which covers the toes and midfoot region; the heel section (quarter) is absent.

Sandalettes and mules are fashion variants of the sandal and slipper respectively. The heel of the sandalette, for example, is generally slightly higher than in the sandal. In mules the vamp is also generally discontinuous, with the result that parts of the toe region are open as with sandals.

The upper is referred to as closed if it rises continuously from the edge of the entire shoe bottom. Shoes with closed uppers include the low shoe (Fig. 5) in which the top line of the upper rises to below the malleolus; the ankle boot (high shoe), whose upper ends above the malleolus; the half-boot which rises to mid-calf height; and the knee boot which accommodates the full height of the calf.

Almost without exception, orthopedic footwear is made with closed uppers only, and generally in the Derby style.

The upper may be provided with various *types of fastening*. A casual shoe (or loafer) has no fastening at all. Buckles are fastened with leather straps and the low shoe most common in orthopedic use is fastened with laces.

1.3 Properly Fitting Footwear

The shoe "should safeguard the foot from harmful external factors such as dirt, dust, moisture and cold, and should afford protection against injury" (KRAUS, 1973). However, footwear should also be consistent with the varied functions which the foot is called upon to perform. For example, a mountaineering boot will be designed differently from a ballet shoe. One single shoe shape or type cannot possibly cater for the vast range of all possible mechanical and functional stresses placed on the human foot. Nevertheless, some general guidelines can be drawn up to ensure that footwear fits properly.

Obviously, *the shoe must not be too short*: in other words, it should not cause the toes to jar painfully against the toe-end of the shoe. It should be remembered in this context that the longitudinal arch of the foot flattens and lengthens during the initial phase of rollover. These factors are compensated for by making the shoe slightly too long. This extra length (generally approximately 1.5 cm or 0.6 inches measured with the foot in the non-load-bearing position) also allows a child's foot space to grow.

The forward shearing movement of the foot is counteracted by ensuring that *the shoe fits snugly* at the level of the calcaneocuboid joint (the insole may be raised slightly under the sustentaculum tali) and that the upper grips the metatarsal region well.

Shoes which are too short restrict the movement of the toes and impair the function of the foot. This fact must be taken into account even at the stage of insole construction. Over the years several insole construction methods have been elaborated, but these cannot be discussed here. Nevertheless, it is generally true that the smaller the foot, the more room the toes require. In infants this results in the *straight ray position* in which the midlines of the metatarsal bones form a continuous straight line with the midlines of the phalanges. In adults, insole construction may permit slight deviation of the great toe and second toe towards the small toe. This applies with ladies' and men's shoes alike. However, the insole is not the only element responsible for ensuring adequate space for the foot inside the shoe; a sufficiently roomy upper is another factor. It can be expecially harmful if the toe-end of the shoe is so narrow that lateral pressure is exerted on the great toe. This not only restricts free movement in the metatarsophalangeal joint, but can also result in valgus deformity. In this context it is important to emphasise that other factors obviously play a crucial role in the evolution of a hallux valgus deformity. However, it would certainly be incorrect to assign no significance at all to a shoe which is excessively narrow and pointed. Daily experience repeatedly confirms this fact.

Even though *shoes which are too large* are generally considered less harmful than shoes which are not wide or long enough, they do have their disadvantages if they are too wide and do not grip the midfoot region properly. Here, too, the toes inevitably impact against the toe-end of the shoe because the foot slides too far forward during toe-off.

The heel of ladies' shoes should not be more than 4 to 4.5 cm (1.6 to 1.8 inches) high if the shoe is genuinely intended for walking purposes and is not designed merely to satisfy the aesthetic dictates of fashion.

Infants' shoes should have *no heel.*

The upper of a low shoe should not be so high as to cover the malleolus. There should be a slight gap between the lower malleolar prominence and the top line of the upper during standing. There will then be no contact between the two as a result of tilting movements during walking.

The material from which the sole is made should be hard and elastic and not yield too readily to the pressure of bodyweight. *In infants* and in school-children *the sole should be as flexible as possible* (see below).

It is an old shoemakers' maxim that the height of the toe spring of a new shoe should be the thickness of a pencil.

1.3.1 Functional Footwear for Children

Particular care and attention should be paid to children's footwear. The following points should be noted:

1. Wherever possible, *babies' feet* should remain *unshod*. A mother's fears that her baby might catch cold can be effectively allayed by pointing out that children do not wear gloves all the time.

2. Shoe length should make allowance both for the lengthening of the foot during the mid-stance phase and for a certain growth rate. This generally means that new shoes should extend *about 1.5 cm (0.6 inches) beyond the ends of the toes*.

3. *Pointed shoe styles* must be *avoided* altogether because they invariably exert a harmful bending force on the toes during the years of skeletal growth. When a child is standing, therefore, the leather of the upper should not exert any directional force on the toes. The midline of the first metatarsal bone should form a continuous straight line with the midline of the great toe.

4. *The shoe must be flexible* so that the child's foot can roll over properly and receive the functional stimulus required for its development. Upper stiffeners, especially in the rear part of the shoe, are to be deplored in children's footwear.

5. Given the increased need for the child's foot to roll over, it follows that the smaller the child, *the lower the ideal heel*. The shoe of the pre-walker and the toddler has no heel.

6. The question of the correct material for children's footwear is particularly important. The *upper* should always be made of *leather* because this best meets the increased need of the child's foot for materials which breathe. Ideally, the outsole should also be made of leather. From the middle years of childhood onwards there is virtually no objection to non-slip plastic soles provided that flexibility is preserved.

Patent leather shoes for children not only betray a certain misguided taste, but are also not to be recommended because the upper is not sufficiently pliable and does not permit the passage of water vapour. This is a particular drawback with children's feet because they normally tend to perspire rather more than adults' feet. For this reason, too, *sandals* are recommended *in summer*.

2 The Mechanics
of the Ankle Joint

In the provision of orthopedic footwear, there are two biomechanical factors which are of major importance and which both have their origin in the concept of the foot as a lever:

1. The foot as a two-armed lever.
2. The ratio between the force arm and the resistance arm during the toe-off phase.

2.1 Lever Actions in the Foot

The question as to whether the foot functions as a single-armed or two-armed lever would really be of only theoretical significance had the important practical terms *"anterior lever"* and *"posterior lever"* (which presuppose a two-armed lever system) not become so firmly entrenched in orthopedic shoe technology. For practical reasons, these concepts have become indispensable because they help us to understand certain shoe technology principles. The action of many shoe components and orthopedic elements (the heel, for example) is in fact due predominantly to their effect on this two-armed lever principle.

During ambulation the foot functions alternately as a two-armed and single-armed lever with smooth transition from one to the other. During the swing phase, for example, it should be regarded as a two-armed lever: the foot moves into dorsiflexion from plantar flexion mainly as a result of the force exerted by the pretibial muscles (F_2) and in concert with the yielding force of the calf muscles (F_1) (Fig. 6). During this process, the application points for F_1 and F_2 are on opposite sides of the fulcrum force F_z, thus creating the physical conditions which define a two-armed lever. The force F_z is equivalent to but operates in an opposite direction to the resultant of forces F_1 and F_2. This resultant F_z is

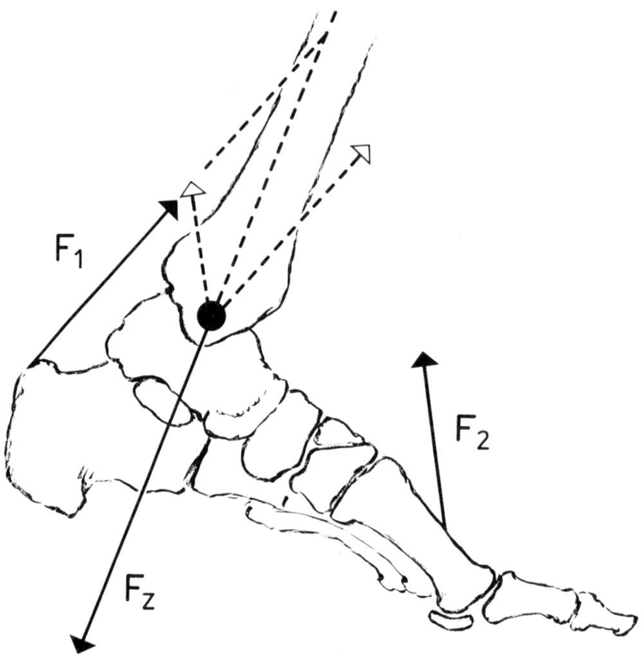

Fig. 6. The foot as a two-armed lever during the swing phase. F_1 plantar flexion force, F_2 dorsiflexion force, F_z fulcrum

thought of as acting at the axis (of the ankle joint). The theoretical importance of the swing phase in the act of walking has undoubtedly been underestimated on occasion. However, its principal role is to create the conditions necessary for the correct and undisturbed toe-off phase during foot contact with the ground. The manner in which the foot is set down is determined during the non-load-bearing phase of walking.

2.1.1 Biomechanics during the Toe-off Phase

During the toe-off phase the foot functions almost exclusively as a single-armed lever (Fig. 7). At heel contact the apex of the plantar surface of the calcaneus becomes the axis. This axis then moves forward very slightly and the entire foot rotates around it. At heel-rise the axis is then transferred to the ball of the foot. In the interim, during the brief period of foot-flat, it would again be legitimate to speak of the foot as a two-armed lever whose anterior arm (a) ex-

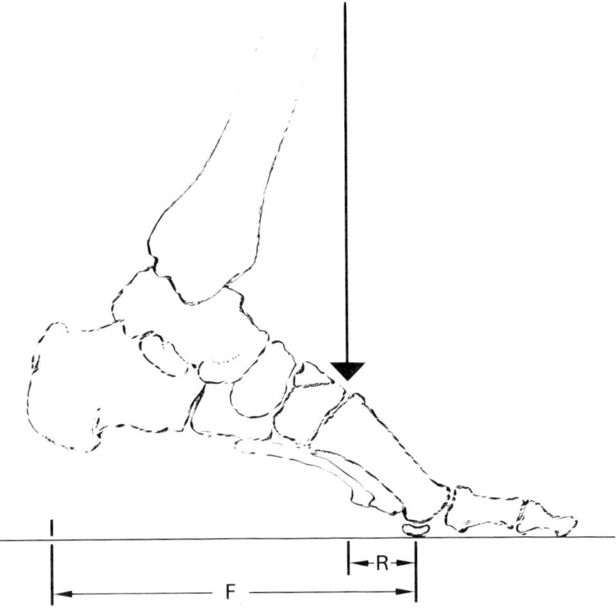

Fig. 7. The foot as a single-armed lever. F force arm, R resistance arm

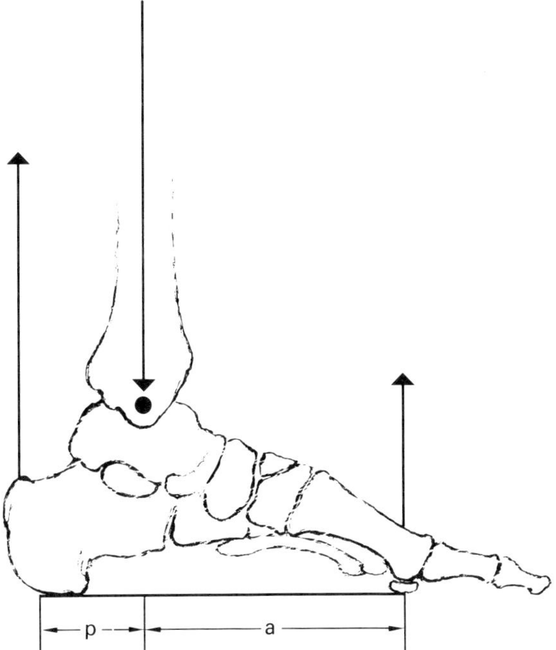

Fig. 8. The foot as a two-armed lever during the stance phase. a anterior lever, p posterior lever

tends between the ankle joint and the ball of the foot, and whose posterior arm (p) reaches from the ankle joint to the apex of the plantar surface of the calcaneus (Fig. 8). Here, too, the resultants of the applied moments are briefly on opposite sides of the fulcrum point.

Certain authorities sometimes betray a measure of illogicality in this area. On a theoretical level, with regard to the provision of orthopedic footwear, they consider the foot (either absolutely or predominantly) as a single-armed lever because this is more correct physics, but they persist simultaneously in referring to an anterior and a posterior lever because this is more consistent with practical requirements.

Alternation between the single- and two-armed lever during walking occurs rapidly and continuously throughout the gait cycle. Footwear can never take full account of these theoretical considerations because, in physicomechanical terms, many orthopedic shoe elements tend to function rather rigidly and without continuity in the individual phases of the gait cycle. This also applies with regard to their influence on anterior or posterior lever action. Nevertheless, application of the principle of the anterior or posterior lever with reference to orthopedic footwear has proved especially effective, not least perhaps because it offers the advantage of simplicity.

2.2 Force and Resistance Arms in the Foot

Similarly, the distinction between the force arm and the resistance arm in the foot is of certain practical importance in the provision of orthopedic footwear. From heel-rise until the end of toe-off, the force arm extends approximately from the Achilles tendon attachment to the ball of the foot, while the resistance arm is the section between the ball of the foot and the gravity line of the body. Normally, this gravity line advances with forward body lean during the toe-off phase. The ratio between the force arm and the resistance arm increases, and the force required to raise the rear part of the foot diminishes continuously during forward propulsion (because force × force arm = resistance × resistance arm). Thus, a raised shoe heel slightly reduces the increased force required initially for the calf muscles to induce heel-rise because the foot is already in the "easier" position of plantar flexion. Clearly, this is only the case when the forward lean of the body is undisturbed.

To summarise: There is a continuing need in the provision of orthopedic footwear to differentiate between an anterior and a posterior lever arm. During the stance phase the posterior arm extends from the apex of the plantar surface of the calcaneus to a point vertically beneath the ankle joint, while the anterior arm extends from this same point to the plantar surface of the ball of the foot. The length relationships between the two lever arms vary with the anatomical position of the foot (e. g. the equinus foot). In this particular case, the anterior arm would be shorter than the posterior arm during standing, and this would need to be taken into account in the provision of appropriate footwear.

3 Orthopedic Elements: Actions and Indications

An orthopedic element is a device which is fitted to a shoe in order to fulfil a specific functional task. This may be to lend support, to compensate for areas of unevenness, to assist rollover, to inhibit or promote movement, to absorb shock, to correct a deformity or to relieve pressure. Any shoe component, usually exaggerated or remodelled in some way, may become an orthopedic element if it is fitted or re-shaped to fulfil one of these functions. Then there are additional elements which are not found in normal shoes, e.g. stiffeners or orthopedic bars.

3.1 Insole

In the very broadest terms, the insole performs three functions: it determines the shape of the entire shoe on a horizontal plane with the prime purpose of ensuring adequate toe space; it has a certain moisture-absorbing capacity to take up foot perspiration; and it should ensure that the foot does not slide about inside the shoe.

In orthopedic footwear these insole functions assume a somewhat subordinate role because a loose moulded insole support (see below) generally forms the interface between foot and shoe. In cases where a loose moulded insole support is not required, however, the following additional elements may be fitted to the insole (although they may equally be fitted to a loose moulded insole).

3.1.1 Metatarsal Pad (Splayfoot Pad)

This is an elastic pad of varying height positioned centrally on the insole immediately behind the metatarsal heads, rising steeply anteriorly and tapering gently posteriorly (Fig. 9). Under no circumstances should the pad ever be positioned beneath the metatarsal heads themselves because this would cause painful pressure discomfort. This device is used to raise the transverse arch in splayfoot deformity. It is referred to as a splayfoot pad when it is made of elas-

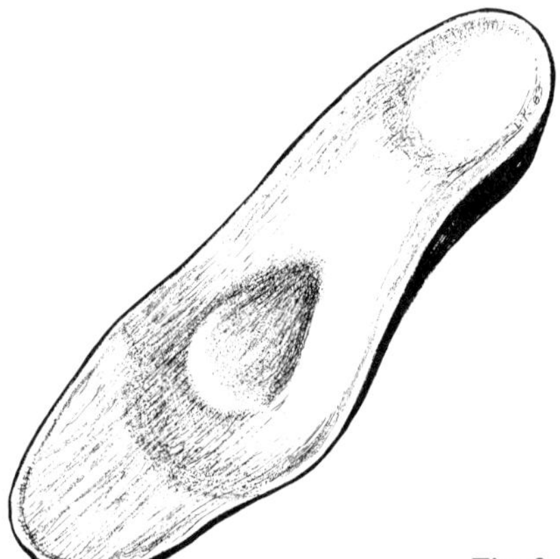

Fig. 9. Metatarsal pad (splayfoot pad)

tic material, and as a metatarsal pad in the narrower sense if the elevation is hard and unyielding, as is the case with metal inserts. It is designed to raise the transverse arch only slightly and should not cause pain. On a practical note, the metatarsal pad is usually inserted between the insole proper and the whole-length sock (see above).

3.1.2 Pressure-Relieving Material

A particularly soft material (foam rubber or similar) is used to relieve pressure. This is inserted into the insole directly underneath painful areas on the plantar surface of the foot, e.g. tender scars, plantar warts or tender bony prominences. In addition, other pressure-bearing areas of the insole may be built up using elastic material, thus affording further relief to the sensitive areas of the sole.

3.1.3 Moulded Insole

A moulded insole is one which has been specially contoured to conform exactly to the weight-bearing surfaces at the heel and ball areas of the foot and, where appropriate, to take account of painful plantar prominences. *It is designed to distribute weight-bearing* over as extensive an insole surface area as possible, thus affording relief to several painful areas at once. However, the advantage of alleviating pain by distributing ground reactive force over a larger area of insole is offset by the *increased energy expended on walking.* The increased ground contact area causes the patient to assume a rather flat-footed, stamping gait. A good moulded insole thus largely inhibits the elastic rollover of the foot which should be characterised by the alternate flattening and raising of the arch during the individual phases of the gait cycle. A moulded insole which is not too hard can make walking endurable or even possible again for the first time for rheumatoid arthritis patients with severely deformed and sensitive feet. Similarly, a moulded insole provides the soft padding necessary for the tender feet of patients with peripheral vascular disease.

3.1.4 Toe Grip Bar

This is a ridge-like elevation which runs transversely across the top of the insole between the contact surfaces at the toes and the ball of the foot (Fig. 10). It

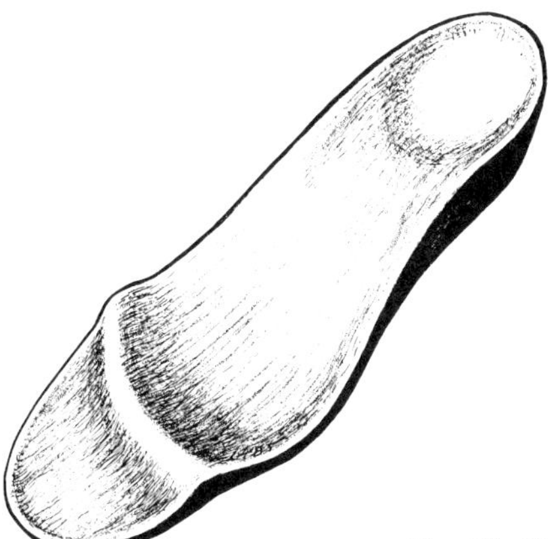

Fig. 10. Toe grip bar

is designed to prevent the foot from sliding forward excessively inside the shoe during the strike phase. It is indicated primarily in contracted equinus foot or to support the foot in equinus when compensating for leg inequality.

3.2 Compensatory Support (Cork Inlay) and Stepped Insole

3.2.1 Compensatory Support (Cork Inlay)

This is a type of insert which is placed between the insole and the plantar surface of the foot. All the orthopedic elements mentioned so far in connection with the insole can be incorporated into a compensatory support. Orthopedic bars (see below) or stiffeners can also be fitted. Virtually all orthopedic shoes are made with this type of compensatory support. The main advantage of this system is that minor foot deformities can be compensated for speedily and repairs can be effected easily without having to re-design the entire shoe. While the compensatory support should also be removable, it should not slip around inside the shoe.

This type of support is required in all cases where the insole does not provide adequate union between the sole of the foot and the shoe bottom. Foot deformities and leg length inequality are almost automatic indications for a compensatory support of this kind.

Although materials of varying elasticity are used, the cushion of the support, covered with sock-lining leather, was at one time (and is occasionally still) made of cork – hence the alternative name cork inlay.

The distinction between a compensatory support and an internal shoe (see below) is uncomplicated and straightforward in that the internal shoe always also has a type of upper, possibly with the associated orthopedic elements, with the result that occasionally it can even be worn inside a retail shoe. This is not so with a compensatory support.

3.2.2 Stepped Insole

The Berlakovits stepped insole is a special type of compensatory support (Fig. 11). The underlying principle is that instead of supporting the plantar deformity over the largest possible contact surface, the stepped insole seeks to *correct pressure distribution.* This is achieved by supporting the sole of the foot in a stepped fashion. These steps are intended not merely to relieve the pressure on painful plantar regions, but also to correct individual foot joints. An additional functional principle underlying the stepped insole is that it can act *to conserve energy.* If an ordinary insole or compensatory support is fitted to

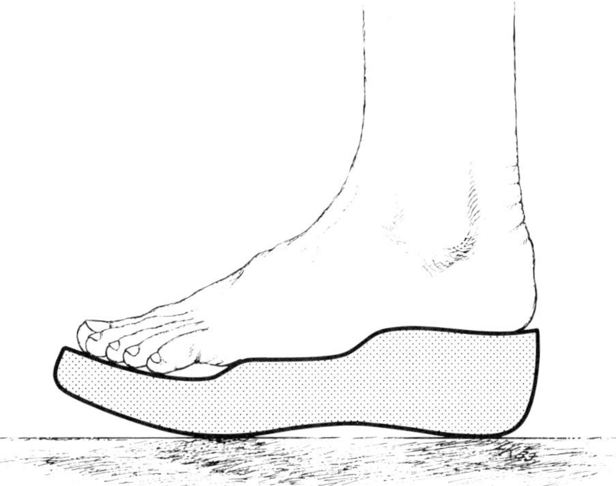

Fig. 11. Berlakovits stepped insole (as compensatory support)

conform perfectly to the anatomical shape of the plantar surface of the foot (a universal desideratum even a few decades ago), the foot becomes largely deprived of its ability to undergo elastic shape change, rather similar to the sensation of running in sand. The patient's gait becomes ponderous as in pronounced pes planus. The frequent consequences of this are foot pain and lower-leg discomfort. It is not without good reason that the normal foot has three weight-bearing points and does not simply present an absolutely flat plantar surface. It would be irresponsible to prescribe a moulded insole (the opposite of a stepped insole) in the absence of specific indications.

In clubfoot, for example, the stepped insole raises the anterior part of the calcaneus on a step to bring it out of equinus. There is an additional stepped support directly behind the first to fifth metatarsal heads, and especially behind the fifth metatarsal head. This causes the plantar aponeurosis and the digital flexor tendons to tense. The longitudinal arch is thus strictly excluded from support. Pressure relief must of course be afforded to painful plantar regions. This exerts a corrective effect on claw toes and on the exaggeratedly high longitudinal arch in pes cavus. The principal indications for a stepped insole are therefore clubfoot, pes cavus and claw toes.

Although the stepped insole is commonly fashioned as a loose compensatory support, its effectiveness is maximised when the steps are incorporated directly into the regular insole because this gives a more intimate functional union between the orthopedic element and the orthopedic shoe. Conversely, with the stepped insole in particular, further minor corrections after manufacture and a wearing-in period may be necessary. Sometimes it is even debatable whether the patient will ever become accustomed to it. This is especially true in cases where there is to be perfect and absolutely painless transfer of step pressure to the sole of the foot. In such cases, it is more advisable and cheaper to have a compensatory support which can be readily removed from the shoe and corrected individually than to have a built-in element.

3.3 Outsole and Orthopedic Bars

In functional terms the outsole is closely linked with the shoe heel. The fitting of any orthopedic element to the outsole must therefore always take the heel into account.

3.3.1 Outsole Thickness

A relatively thick outsole is of prime importance in shoes intended to correct leg inequality. The need for a corresponding increase in heel height is self-evident in such cases.

A relatively thin outsole is useful in correcting supination with an orthopedic shoe and occasionally, for example, in clubfoot. In such cases, a thicker outsole would be inappropriate because the shoe invariably displays particularly marked lateral wear. Consequently, the force counteracting supination is rapidly lost over the course of time, and the shoe is sent in too late for outsole replacement because the patient does not always recognise the wear on the functional element soon enough.

3.3.2 Medial or Lateral Wedging

These wedges should only be fitted to the orthopedic shoe in exceptional circumstances because the corrective effects potentially achieved by raising the rim of the sole in this way can be achieved more easily and effectively by using a compensatory support. The purpose of wedging is to alter the position of the entire foot to bring about supination (medial wedging) or pronation (lateral wedging); generally this means that the heel also has to be wedged on one side. As a modification to a retail shoe, this may be appropriate following ligament injuries or to compensate for an exostosis at the base of the proximal phalanx of the hallux and projecting beneath the level of the sole (in this case, in association with an appropriate insert). Similarly, pronation contraction of the forefoot in pes equinoexcavatus can also be corrected by lateral wedging. This has a beneficial effect on pain beneath the second metatarsal head. However, medial wedging to correct infantile genu valgum is somewhat outmoded, not simply because it flattens the arch of the foot but also because the elevation of the medial edge of the foot sets the ankle and subtalar joints at an unphysiologically oblique angle.

3.3.3 Orthopedic Bars

Orthopedic bars are of major importance and are applied predominantly to the outsole of the shoe *(surface bar)* or between the outsole and the insole *(concealed bar)*. When the bar is fitted to the compensatory support it is referred to as an *internal bar.*

An orthopedic bar is a convex element applied to the bottom of the shoe. Its apex acts as a pivot to assist rollover. The higher the apex, the greater the extent of movement achieved.

Orthopedic bars are intended to substitute for absent movement or to facilitate painful movement. They are thus recommended in cases where joints are stiff or irritated. Since the apex of the bar acts as a pivot, it should be positioned at right angles to the direction of movement. Here, too, care should be taken *to ensure appropriate heel compensation.* Any orthopedic bar, with the exception of the toe bar, raises the forefoot by comparison with the heel. Consequently, apart from certain exceptional circumstances where such an effect might be desirable, the shoe heel should always be raised on both sides in a manner consistent with the elevation produced by the orthopedic bar.

The effectiveness of the orthopedic bar also depends on the shoe bottom no longer possessing significant flexibility. This applies most particularly when the shoe is worn over an extended period. There is also a constant danger that the bar (which has to bear the entire groundward pressure of the bodyweight on a relatively small area) may be "trodden into the shoe" over the course of time (KRAUS, 1973). For this reason, the shoe bottom should usually also be *reinforced,* preferably with a steel plate. Needless to say, the apex of the bar will be worn down with time and consequently, wear should be checked at frequent and regular intervals.

A major *disadvantage* with all orthopedic bars (not merely with those applied to the actual outsole) is that the elevation and increased thickness between the sole of the foot and the ground deprive the foot of the sensation of ground contact and hence of a certain degree of steadiness during walking. The reduction in gait steadiness is critically intensified by the fact that the apex of the rocker bar or metatarsal bar is placed behind the physiological transverse axis of the foot which follows the line of the metatarsal heads. This reduces the weight-bearing area of the foot which normally extends from the calcaneus to the metatarsal heads. A round-edge heel or raised heel reduces this mechanical weight-bearing area still further, bringing about an additional decline in stance and gait steadiness. Certain neurological disorders, e. g. those associated with ataxia, are thus relative contra-indications for orthopedic bars without any other modifications.

An additional disadvantage is that the shortening of the contralateral limb brought about by orthopedic bar elevation always has to be compensated. The fitting of a bar thus affects the leg which is in fact sound. Finally, it is something of a drawback that certain bars act on adjacent or more remote joints, especially the metatarsal and forefoot joints, and that the shoe bottom needs to be stiffened if full effectiveness is to be achieved. However, stiffening the sole will inevitably abolish any residual physiological movements in the forefoot and metatarsal region which might still have been possible during rollover. For all these reasons, bars should not be prescribed without careful evaluation of the indications and this is why one eminent authority repeatedly "warns against overrating the orthopedic bar technique" (KRAUS, 1973).

The various types of orthopedic bar are distinguished in terms of the position of their apex. The following variations will be discussed in approximately descending order of importance:

1. Rocker bar
2. Metatarsal bar
3. Horseshoe bar
4. L-shaped bar
5. Triangular bar
6. Toe bar
7. Mini-bar

3.3.3.1 Rocker Bar

The apex of the rocker bar lies immediately behind the metatarsophalangeal joints, thus relieving the pressure on the metatarsal heads (Fig. 12). The axis of its apex is at right angles to the direction of walking. The rocker bar is the orthopedic element *par excellence* for functional disorders of the metatarsophalangeal joints and is indicated where mobility is absent, impaired or painful, i. e. primarily in hallux rigidus. In this case, care should be taken to ensure that the apex is located directly underneath the sesamoid bones. A rocker bar together with a heel raise is indicated in patients with leg inequality, and is absolutely essential in patients who have lost toes.

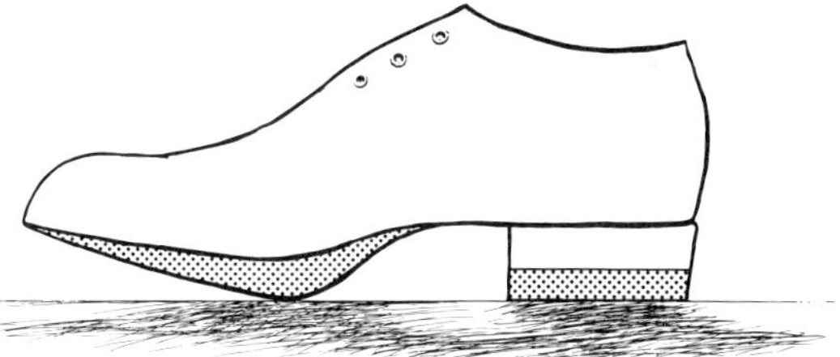

Fig. 12. Rocker bar

3.3.3.2 Metatarsal Bar

The apex of the metatarsal bar lies immediately beneath the metatarsus and is at right angles to the direction of travel (Fig. 13). It is indicated in the following conditions: contraction and painful movement in the tarsus, post-fracture calcaneal deformity and, especially, impaired or potentially impaired ankle joint mobility. The same functions can be fulfilled by a rocker-bottomed wedge heel. The metatarsal bar is prescribed in conjunction with a round-edge heel (buffer heel) to aid rollover, and with a behind-heel float in pes calcaneo-excavatus due to paralysis.

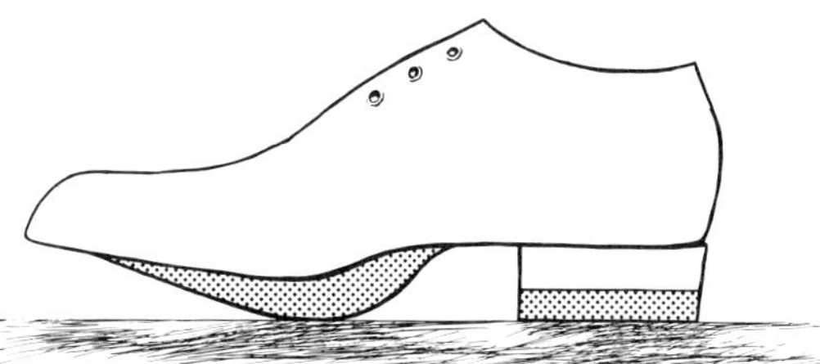

Fig. 13. Metatarsal bar

3.3.3.3 Horseshoe Bar

This bar is U-shaped with two arms (or wings) extending forward on either side of the shoe (Fig. 14). It is used to relieve painful central metatarsal heads, such as are encountered in forefoot contraction and splayfoot.

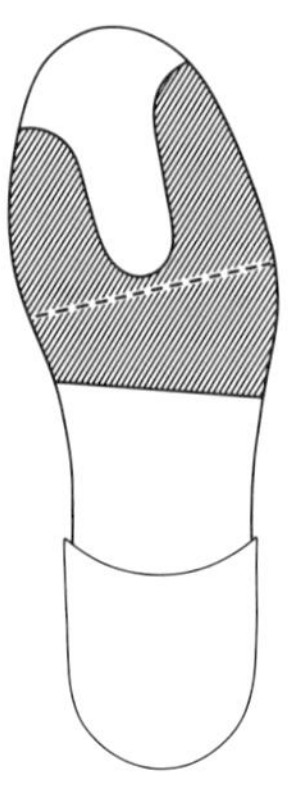

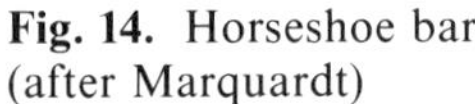

Fig. 14. Horseshoe bar
(after Marquardt)

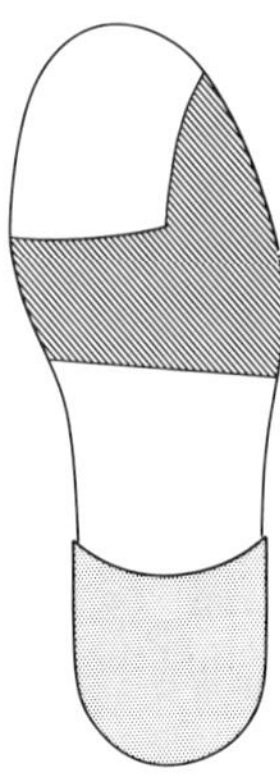

Fig. 15. L-shaped bar

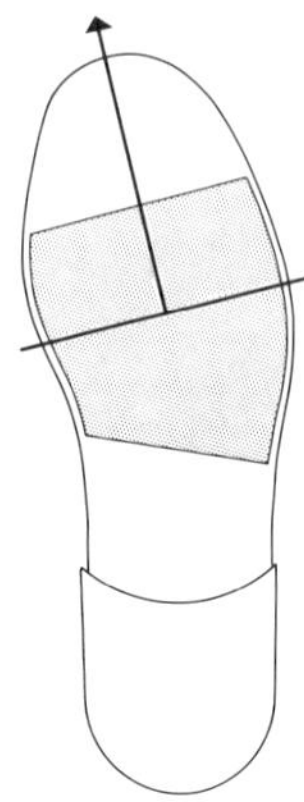

Fig. 16. Triangular bar

3.3.3.4 L-shaped Bar

This is in fact an L-shaped rocker bar with a lateral (or more rarely, a medial) wing projecting anteriorly (Fig. 15). However, its apex is at an oblique angle to the direction of travel. The anterior projection thus influences foot position during the rollover phase by causing detorsion (inward tilting), thus relieving the first to third metatarsal heads. This type of bar is indicated in certain forms of pes cavus and in sesamoid bone irritation.

3.3.3.5 Triangular Bar

This bar is actually not triangular but trapezoidal in shape and is fitted at an oblique angle to the direction of travel (Fig. 16). During rollover it exerts a rotatory force on the foot towards the narrower edge of the bar, either medially or laterally. A case of excessive outward rotation of the foot, for example, would demand that the triangular bar be fitted with the narrower edge positioned medially.

3.3.3.6 Toe Bar

The apex of this bar is placed in front of the metatarsophalangeal joints and is at right angles to the direction of travel (Fig. 17). In mechanical terms, it is not an orthopedic bar, but forms a kind of extension to the anterior lever of the foot. Its function is to lock the knee joint. It is thus indicated preferentially in

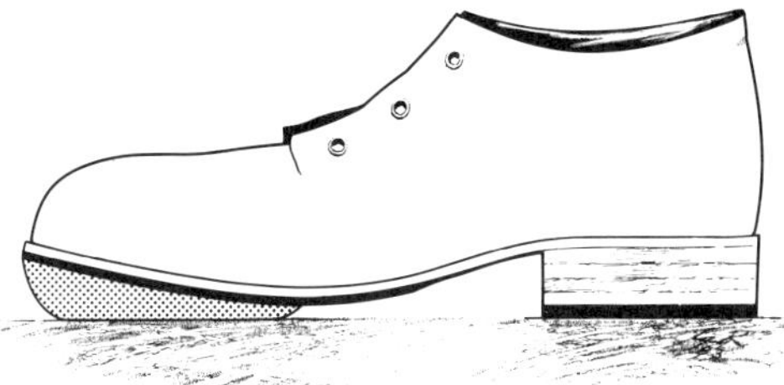

Fig. 17. Toe bar

femoral nerve paralysis (quadriceps weakness). Because this type of bar often causes pain by encouraging arch flattening to a certain extent, the sole of the shoe requires additional stiffening. The locking effect on the knee can be enhanced by fitting the shoe with a low heel, thus bringing the foot further into calcaneus.

3.3.3.7 Mini-Bar

This is an extremely short orthopedic bar with a small radius and narrow base. Its special function is to facilitate rollover but this is achieved at the cost of reduced stance and gait steadiness.

3.3.4 Cradle Shoe

In Henkel's cradle shoe (Fig. 18), the sole, waist and heel constitute both a functional and a physical unit. These three shoe components form a continuous arc, the centre of which should be located approximately at the midpoint of the thigh. This means that, in adults, the rocker height will range from 13 to

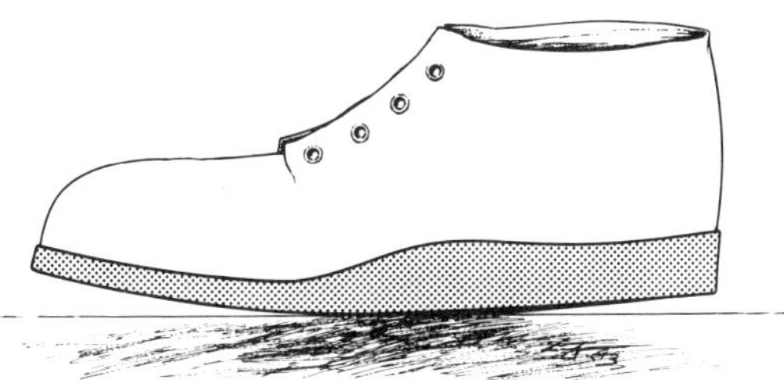

Fig. 18. Henkel's cradle shoe

17 mm (0.5 to 0.7 inches), depending on leg length. Rocker height can be calculated using the following formula:

$$RH = +\sqrt{L^2 + b^2} - L$$

RH = rocker height

L = distance from thigh midpoint to sole of foot

b = half shoe sole length.

In functional terms the heel is in fact fashioned as a (rocker-bottomed) wedge heel: in other words, the dividing line between the sole and the heel is non-existent in the cradle shoe.

This shoe type was designed specifically for the rocker-bottomed foot but might also prove useful in knee stiffness, for example. In this case, the centre of the arc should be located at the midpoint of the hip joint. In the absence of sole stiffeners, the sole of this shoe slightly raises, and thus corrects, the rocker-bottomed longitudinal arch of the foot during rollover. Generally, this model is constructed as a low shoe.

3.4 Special Modifications to the Shoe Bottom

3.4.1 Sole Stiffening

Stiffening the shoe sole has the effect of lengthening the anterior lever of the foot. If this stiffening extends forward beyond the joint line, it will exert a particularly powerful locking action on the knee joint and have the same effect as a toe bar. Sole stiffening is cosmetically more acceptable because the toe spring of the sole is preserved.

In practice, the sole is stiffened by inserting a plate made of steel or some relatively robust plastic material.

Stiffening of the sole is indicated in toe loss and in quadriceps weakness. Stiffening should generally also be prescribed when orthopedic bars are to be fitted in order to prevent the bar from being trodden into the shoe. In forefoot amputation or equinus it is sufficient to stiffen the shoe sole forward as far as, or just short of, the joint line. In such cases, the leading edge of the stiffener compensates for joint line function.

If only the lateral part of the sole stiffener is extended further forward, it exerts an inward rotatory effect and raises the lateral edge of the foot during rollover, similar to the action of a triangular bar. Where the medial part of the shoe stiffener is extended forward, it has an outward rotatory and supinating effect.

3.4.2 Flaring the Sole

A medial or lateral sole flare (floating in or floating out of the sole) discourages valgus or varus movement in the foot and deviation at the knee joint.

A medial sole flare counteracts valgus formation at the knee joint and could be prescribed, for example, in medial ligament flaccidity. This effect would be further intensified by flaring the heel medially (Fig. 19).

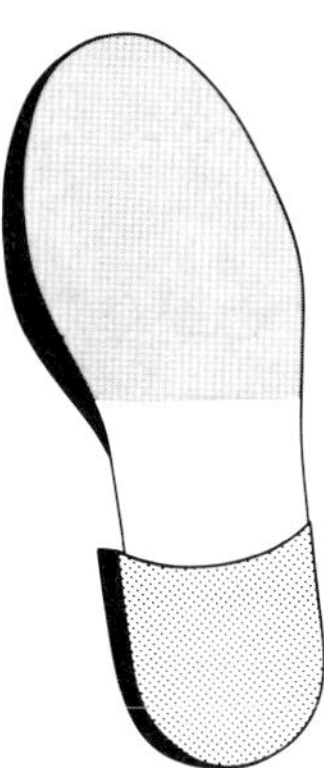

Fig. 19. Medial flare on shoe bottom and heel

3.4.3 Bottom Filler

The bottom filler, the material sandwiched between the insole and the outsole (Fig. 20), is of prime importance in supporting the sole of the foot, particularly in cases where the orthopedic shoe contains no compensatory support. The bottom filler causes pressure to be distributed over the sole of the foot, affords some relief to tender plantar surfaces and restores some potential elastic spring to foot mobility. In sweaty feet, it is mainly the bottom filler which absorbs the moisture. It should thus be made of a material which possesses especially good moisture-absorbing properties. The thickness of the bottom filler

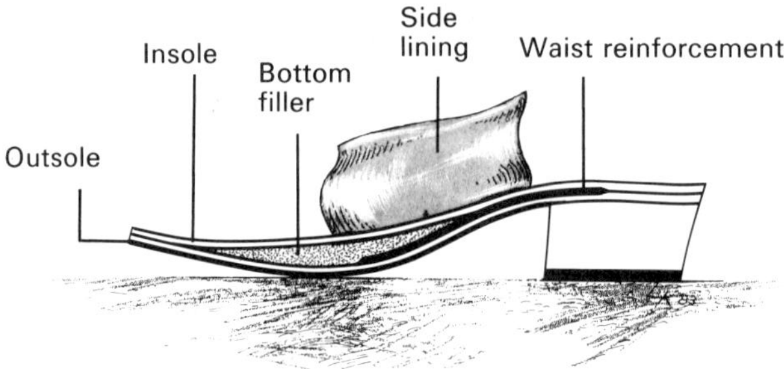

Fig. 20. Shoe bottom with side lining

should be consistent with the welt (the ring-shaped leather strip stitched to the outside of the shoe and serving as a junction between upper and shoe bottom). An overly thick bottom filler will reduce gait elasticity and cause the shoe bottom to bulge after protracted wear, while an excessively thin bottom filler may cause the entire shoe bottom to become concave. The hardness of the bottom filler is also determined by the tenderness of the plantar surface of the foot and is thus of predominantly technical significance.

3.5 Heel

The effect of the shoe heel as an orthopedic element depends on its height, elasticity and shape. The heel forms an intimate functional unit with the shoe bottom, and in particular with the toe spring. The forward face of the heel is known as the *heel breast.*

3.5.1 Raised Heel

A raised heel moves the gravity line of the body forward in the direction of travel, relieves pressure on the calcaneus and calf muscles and brings increased ground pressure to bear on the forefoot if the calcaneus is not gripped firmly. It also has the effect of shortening stride length and after a protracted time results in the development of lordosis which may ultimately be impossible to correct. This point deserves emphasis because there are those who refuse to accept this view. A raised heel not only makes the shoe look shorter, but also actually reduces the mechanical length of the foot.

A heel should be regarded as raised if it is more than 45 mm (1.8 inches) high in ladies' shoes and more than 35 mm (1.4 inches) high in men's shoes. Mechanically, it has the effect not only of displacing the gravity line forward in the direction of movement during travel, but also of increasing the ratio of the force arm to the resistance arm (see Fig. 9), thus shortening stride length.

For these reasons, a raised heel on an orthopedic shoe is indicated to compensate for leg inequality or in plantar contracture of the ankle joint. Since the raised heel brings the foot further into equinus at the ankle, the movement of this joint is restricted – a beneficial result in cases where mobility is painful. Since it makes less work for the calf muscles during walking, a raised heel may also be of advantage in functional calf pain due to peripheral vascular disease, particularly when a moulded insole is also required to afford soft support to the foot. For mechanical reasons, a raised heel counteracts genu recurvatum and its stride-shortening action can sometimes be utilised to good effect in cases where hip joint mobility is painful.

However, the raised heel is a disadvantage in cases where a pumping action of the calf muscles would be desirable, e.g. in disturbed venous return. Because it tends to encourage lordosis, a raised heel is also inappropriate during pregnancy because the centre of gravity of the body is displaced forward in any case as the pregnancy becomes more advanced. Unless the calcaneus is gripped firmly, a raised heel produces overload discomfort in the forefoot in patients with splayfoot.

In the field of shoe construction it is axiomatic that *once a shoe has been made, subsequent raising of the heel is impossible because* the resultant elevation would cause the toe spring of the shoe sole to disappear. Not only would this produce transverse creasing of the upper, but it would also inhibit rollover, quite apart from the fact that such a modification would also place increased stress on the metatarsal heads (Fig. 21).

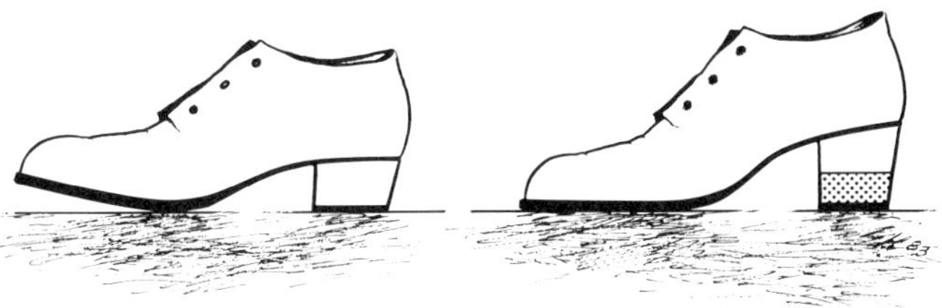

Fig. 21. If the shoe heel only is raised, the toe spring disappears

3.5.2 Low (Flat) Heel

The lower the heel, the more physiological the rollover of the foot and the entire gait cycle. A low heel permits normal stride length and does not diminish the demands placed on the foot and calf muscles. It tends to have a slight locking effect on the knee joint and it does not exacerbate lumbar lordosis. Consequently, the low heel is indicated whenever venous return needs to be stimulated. It is especially recommended during pregnancy because it does not intensify lordosis, and it may even be indicated in quadriceps weakness (together with a toe bar or a stiffened sole, where appropriate).

However, the low heel is contra-indicated in cases where the tarsal or ankle joints are painful on movement, in excessively painful peripheral vascular disorders, in pain under the calcaneus during toe-off and in genu recurvatum which the musculature is unable to stabilise with sufficient firmness. The low heel should also preferably be avoided in conditions where the hip joints are painful on movement.

3.5.3 Behind-Heel Float

This is a type of heel which is floated out posteriorly, thus modifying the ratio of resistance arm to force arm in favour of the force arm by lengthening the posterior lever of the foot (see Fig. 40). The behind-heel float thus causes plantar flexion during toe-off and counteracts dorsiflexion. This action can be further enhanced by advancing the position of the calcaneus inside the shoe by inserting material between its posterior surface and the heel counter. Care should also be taken here to ensure that the calcaneus is still able to move backwards slightly. Apart from causing plantar flexion, a behind-heel float also acts to flatten the longitudinal arch of the foot. It should be remembered that this modification should always be prescribed in conjunction with a metatarsal bar (see Fig. 40).

The behind-heel float is indicated in tibial nerve paralysis, a condition in which tibial muscle force totally overwhelms the plantar-flexing muscles of the calf.

3.5.4 Extended Heel and Wedge Heel

An extended heel is one which is elongated anteriorly across its entire width, and a wedge heel is one which is projected forward as far as the break of the

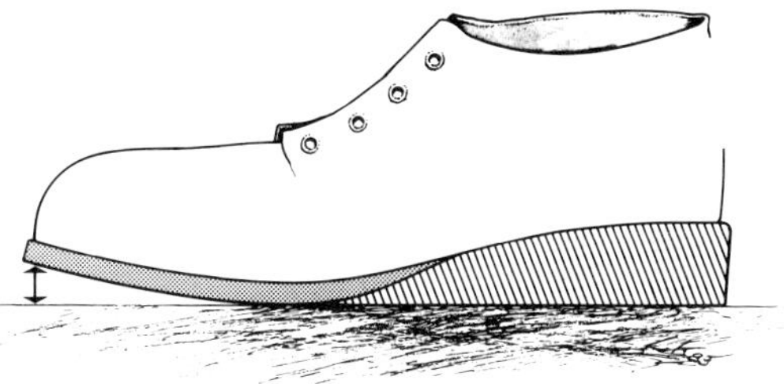

Fig. 22. Wedge heel ($\updownarrow$ toe spring)

shoe (Fig. 22) and thus fills the entire waist of the shoe. Both heel types reduce the flexibility of the shoe and thus act to stabilise the waist. They also increase the area of contact between the shoe bottom and the underlying surface.

Extended heels and wedge heels are indicated in cases where the shoe waist needs to be stabilised, e. g. in contracted and severely deformed pes planovalgus. The extended heel is one of the salient features of the rigid rocker-sole shoe (see 5.2.1), and the central element of the continuous sole of the cradle shoe is, in functional terms, part of a wedge heel, although cradle-shaped in this particular case.

3.5.5 Heel with Central Waist Support

This heel type is characterised by a support which extends forward across the central part of the waist only (Fig. 23). It lends greater elastic stability to the shoe waist and enlarges the contact surface with the ground. It fulfils approximately the same function as the extended heel but is in fact rarely prescribed. Its chief significance is to increase the non-slip properties of the shoe.

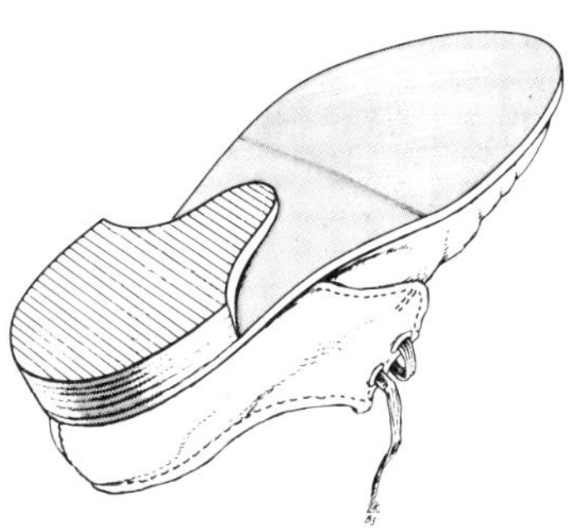

Fig. 23. Heel with central waist support

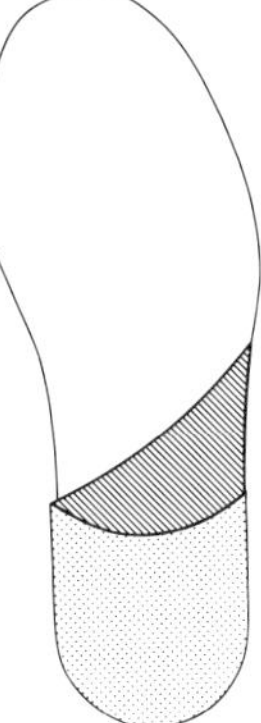

Fig. 24. Thomas heel

3.5.6 Thomas Heel

This type of heel has an anterior triangular extension, lateral or medial, into the waist of the shoe (Fig. 24). Its principal function is to stabilise the shoe waist where it is anticipated that this might collapse under stress on one side, e.g. where the longitudinal arch of the foot is under a relatively heavy load.

3.5.7 Laterally or Medially Displaced Heel

With this heel type, one side is significantly displaced laterally or medially while the opposite side is moved more towards the midpoint of the heel (Fig. 25). This modification is intended to discourage varus or valgus formation, e.g. in flaccidity of the medial ankle ligaments with a tendency to tilt due to medial displacement. Conversely, there is always the danger on uneven surfaces that the shoe will twist in the opposite direction more easily.

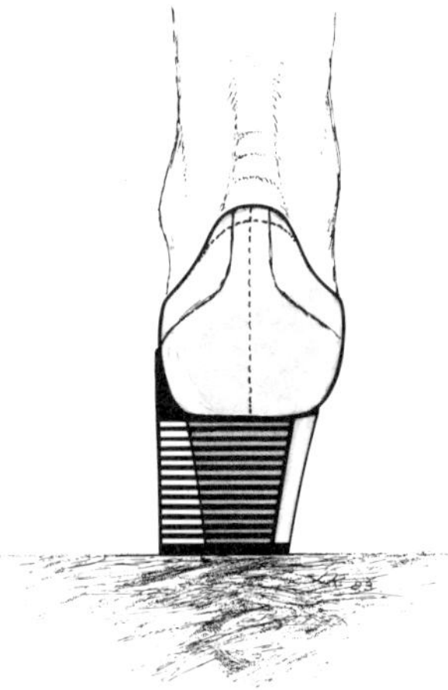

Fig. 25. Heel displaced laterally

3.5.8 Ball Heel

As the name implies, this heel is ball-shaped. It exerts an active rather than a passive corrective effect and is actually an exercise heel used to strengthen the muscles in pes planovalgus in infancy, in which case the crown of the curvature is displaced slightly medially. The ball heel is in fact never prescribed with an orthopedic shoe, but exclusively as a modification to a retail shoe. In such circumstances, however, it should always be combined with an insert with a lateral flange, and as a general principle the calcaneus should be well supported and the heel as a whole should be as low as possible.

3.5.9 Buffer Heel and Round-Edge Heel

Both heel types were designed to absorb compressive forces during heelstrike and to facilitate rollover of the shoe during the heel-strike phase. The round-edge heel is tapered posteriorly so that, when the shoe is standing on a flat surface, about one-third to one-half of the heel at the back is not in contact with the ground (Fig. 26). The buffer heel is made of especially shock-absorb-

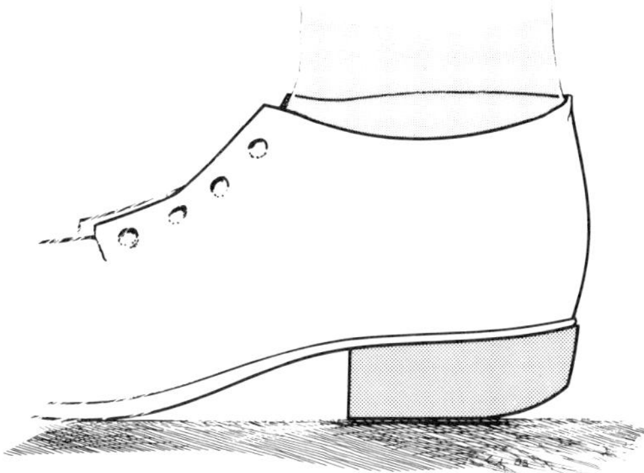

Fig. 26. Round-edge heel

ent material and, like the round-edge heel, generally facilitates rollover (Fig. 27). However, it has the advantage over the round-edge heel that it is more slip-resistant. Currently, therefore, the round-edge heel is prescribed only rarely, and usually when it is necessary to prevent bending at the knee, because the buffer heel has a slightly greater knee-bending effect.

The round-edge heel shortens the resistance arm by comparison with the force arm. A similar effect is achieved as a result of the compressibility of the buffer heel. Not only is impact absorbed during heel-strike but, due to the posterior lever arm becoming shorter, less effort is required of the muscles which dorsiflex the foot.

For this reason, the buffer heel (or round-edge heel) is indicated whenever impact energy on heel-strike needs to be converted into deformation energy,

e. g. in painful heel-strike, in degenerative and painful changes in the knee and hip joints, and in dorsiflexor weakness to facilitate rollover. The rigid rockersole shoe has one or other of these heel types almost by definition.

The hardness of the buffer heel depends on the patient's bodyweight and the clinical diagnosis. Heavier patients require a harder heel. Conversely, a softer modification is indicated in spinal disorders and in patients with hip and knee prostheses.

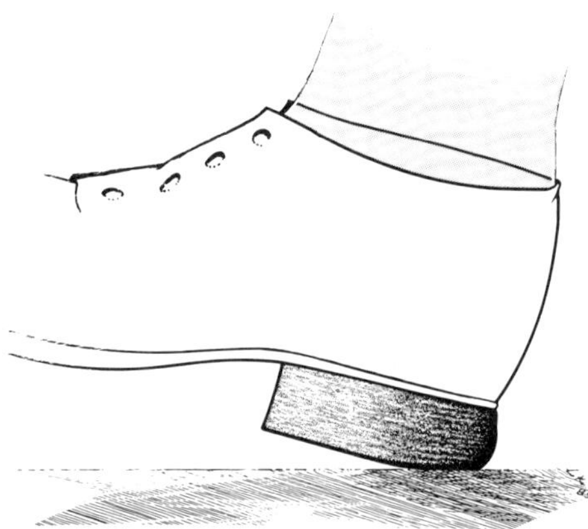

Fig. 27. Buffer heel

3.6 Waist

Although it is known that, for a physiological gait, the shoe waist should be as elastic as possible so as not to inhibit the normal play of movement of the foot in all directions, pathological factors very often dictate that the waist be stiffened, with the result that such movement is largely prevented. Waist stiffening is necessary especially in cases where stiffening elements are also incorporated into the shoe upper. Similarly, any compensatory support necessitates stiffening of the waist, as do measures to correct leg inequality, partial foot loss and, generally, equinus. It is therefore not absolutely necessary to specify waist stiffening as such in the orthopedic shoe prescription. It may also be mentioned that very few retail shoes nowadays do not incorporate a stiffened waist.

3.7 Upper with Stiffeners and Reinforced Tongue

The special functional effect of the upper is determined by its height, its mode of fastening and the manner in which it is reinforced or stiffened.

A normal laced ankle boot (high shoe) is approximately 14 cm (5.6 inches) high, measured above the medial malleolus. In foot paralysis, and where cover for an internal shoe is required, higher uppers may be necessary, and in paralysis these may be as much as 25 cm (10 inches) high.

3.7.1 Internal Fastening

This is an especially effective means of fixing the foot in position. The internal fastener is fashioned as a fairly broad leather strap assembly attached to the back part of the shoe bottom and passed round a wide area of the metatarsus.

3.7.2 Eisenmann Strap

This strap (Fig. 28) performs the same function as the internal fastener. It too is attached between the upper and the shoe bottom and passes round the meta-

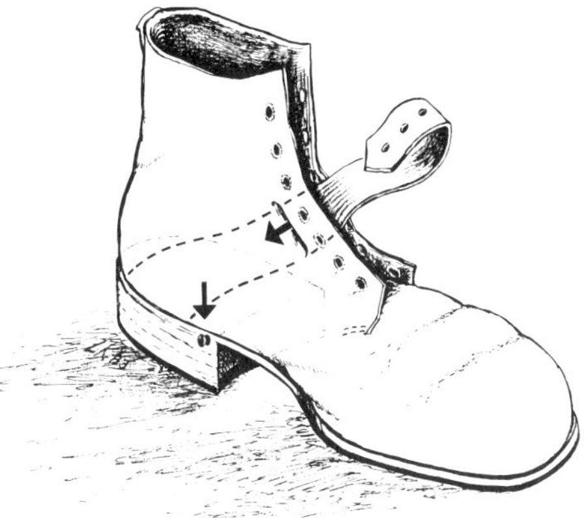

Fig. 28. Eisenmann strap

tarsus. Unlike the internal fastener, however, the Eisenmann strap is not only narrower, but is also fed out from inside the shoe through a slit near the eyelet facing and is attached again to the shoe bottom on the outside.

3.7.3 Upper Reinforcement

The upper may be reinforced with boot loops or leather side pieces. The boot loop is designed to assist the wearer in pulling the shoe on (for example, where the foot is stiff) and is a smooth leather strap attached inside the shoe in front of the back seam.

Leather side pieces merely serve to reinforce the lining of the upper and are used mainly in appliance shoes.

3.7.4 Upper Stiffening

Stiffening of the upper needs to be differentiated from reinforcement of the upper. Stiffening of the upper is achieved using stiffeners (and side linings) which are generally inserted between the lining and the outside leather and serve to protect the foot (industrial footwear) or to inhibit movement (see Fig. 20). Where stiffeners have to be particularly robust, they are made of fibre-glass reinforced casting resin or, for protective functions, of metal. Depending on their location, they are referred to as toe caps or heel counters.

The *toe cap* serves to stiffen the upper or preserve the shape of the toe-end of the shoe (see Fig. 2). It is indicated to protect the toes from injury or – usually as an extended toe cap which reaches back beyond the metatarsophalangeal joints – to provide additional stiffening for the front part of the shoe when the toes or forefoot have been lost.

Heel counters are of outstanding importance in orthopedic terms because they are the major stabilising and controlling element in the orthopedic shoe.

The following different types of heel counter are found:

1. Extended lateral or medial heel counter
2. Lateral or medial ankle stiffener (support counter)
3. High stiffener to counteract peroneal nerve paralysis
4. High ankle stiffener (Berlin stiffener)

3.7.4.1 Extended Lateral or Medial Heel Counter

This is a stiffening element which extends forward to stiffen the shoe laterally or medially. It stabilises the shoe against sideways movement, for example, in clubfoot which is still partially susceptible to passive correction. In this case, the heel counter extends forward laterally as far as the metatarsophalangeal joints (Fig. 29).

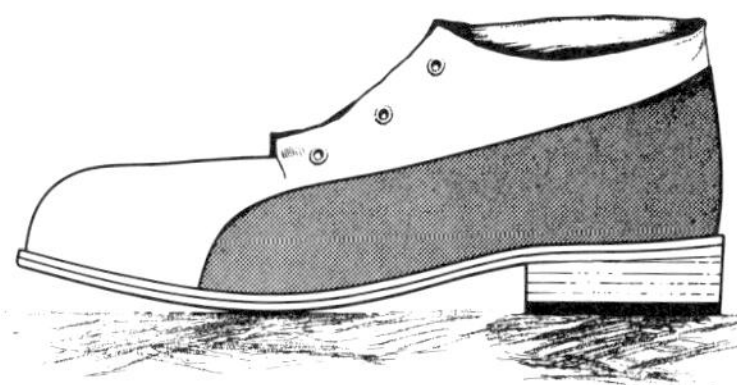

Fig. 29. Heel counter extended forward medially (or laterally)

3.7.4.2 Ankle Support Counter

This extends forward from the back of the shoe around the lateral or medial malleolus and is intended to discourage hindfoot supination and pronation respectively.

3.7.4.3 High Stiffener to Counteract Peroneal Nerve Paralysis

The high peroneal stiffener prevents the ankle joint from moving into plantar flexion and thus inhibits passive foot drop, this being of particular importance at the start of the swing phase (Fig. 30). To enable the lower leg to tilt for-

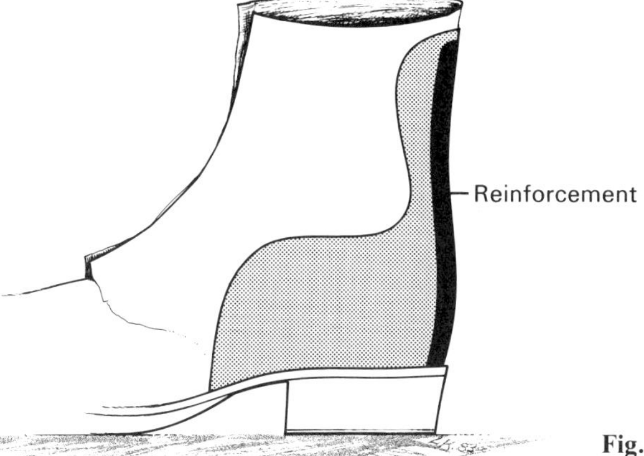

Fig. 30. High stiffener to counteract peroneal nerve paralysis

ward unimpeded during the stance phase, the malleoli must not be immobilised. Starting well back along the shoe sole, the high peroneal stiffener rises broadly at first, tapers to a narrow dorsal bridge at the level of the malleoli and then broadens out again to encase the posterior aspect of the lower leg. The high peroneal stiffener varies in height; for good effectiveness it will be at least 18 cm (7.2 inches) high, and may even be 25 cm (10 inches) high.

3.7.4.4 High Ankle Stiffener (Berlin Stiffener)

This is fashioned in exactly the same way as the high peroneal stiffener, but does not have recesses for the malleoli. Instead, it covers these too and encases about half the girth of the lower leg (Fig. 31).

It is an essential feature of the Rabl rigid rocker-sole shoe (see 5.3.1) and, together with a stiffened tongue (see below), serves to immobilise the ankle joint.

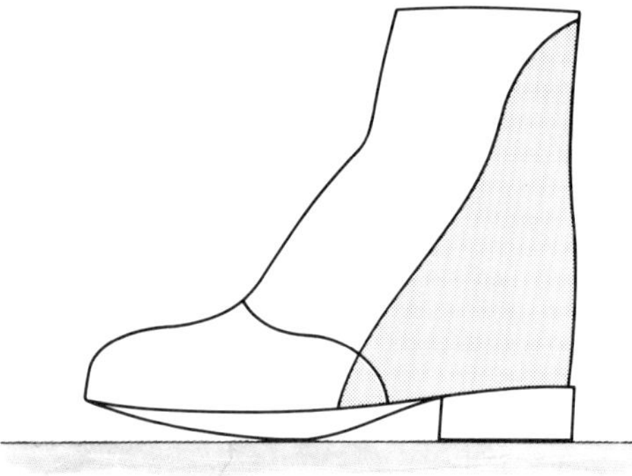

Fig. 31. High ankle stiffener (Berlin stiffener)

3.7.4.5 Stiffened Tongue

This rises from the side of the shoe bottom, passes forward over the ankle joint and embraces the anterior curvature of the lower leg. It is well cushioned in the region of the foot. When stiffening is implemented, precise care should be taken to ensure that the required angle between foot and lower leg is achieved and maintained.

On its own a stiffened tongue is necessary on orthopedic footwear for forefoot amputees. Together with a Berlin stiffener, a stiffened moulded leather tongue immobilises the ankle joint. Because they then form a single functional unit, the Berlin stiffener and stiffened tongue together are also known as a round-ankle stiffener.

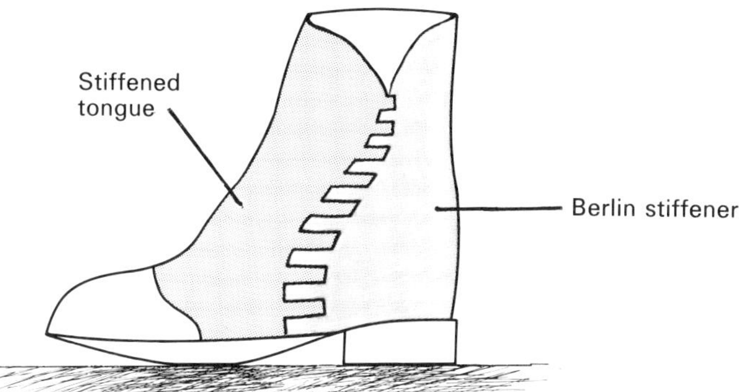

Fig. 32. Round-ankle stiffener

3.7.4.6 Round-Ankle Stiffener

If it is to immobilise the ankle joint with any degree of security, the round-ankle stiffener should be at least 18 cm (7.2 inches) high and fit snugly with the foot and lower leg (Fig. 32).

Tender dorsal areas or painful bony prominences can be cushioned locally by lining the underside of the upper with soft material at appropriate points.

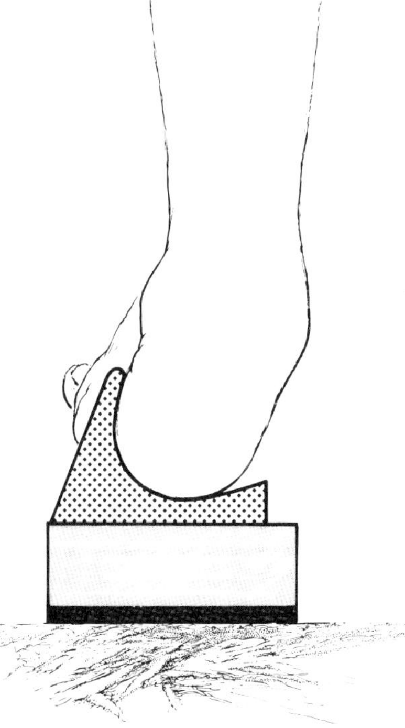

Fig. 33. Supination wedge

This results in an upper which fits snugly and grips the foot well (cushioned areas of upper or cushioned tongue).

3.7.5 Supination Wedge

This is a curved wedge made of sturdy elastic material. Its convex curvature tapers away towards the small toe and the crown of the curvature is located beneath the sustentaculum tali (Fig. 33). It should only extend forward as far as the navicular bone so as not to bring the forefoot into supination too. The supination wedge can be fitted medially in a low shoe. It supinates the hindfoot in pes planovalgus and should actively ensure good torsion here during rollover, a result which is especially beneficial for the muscles of the foot. *Torsion* is the physiological twisting of the foot about its longitudinal axis in such a way that the hindfoot is supinated while the forefoot is pronated (see also 5.1.6.1).

3.8 Internal Shoe

An exact definition of the internal shoe is somewhat elusive. KRAUS (1980) offers the following explanation: "The term 'internal shoe' embraces all orthopedic measures in which individual, orthopedically active elements of the orthopedic shoe are effective but are not integral parts of the outer footwear." This definition is very wide and KRAUS (1980) logically construes the internal shoe as including toe-raising orthoses and tibial plates. The critical point to note is that the internal shoe not only contains at least one active orthopedic element, but also slightly resembles a shoe in appearance and requires a second shoe (very often a retail shoe) as outer cladding in order to function properly. The internal shoe thus consists of an upper and a foot support. Since the internal shoe may often be worn under the sock, the old and succinct "shoe inside a shoe" definition could be slightly misleading.

The main advantage conferred by the internal shoe is that the orthopedically active elements of the shoe are brought into closer proximity to the parts of the foot and lower leg which they are intended to influence, with the result that shearing movements do not actually occur between the shoe and the foot, but between the internal shoe and the outer shoe. There is the additional point that the internal shoe generally offers cosmetic advantages: in particular, the patient is often able to wear retail shoes which are usually more appropriate in fashion terms than custom-made shoes. The internal shoe is also generally lighter in weight.

On the other hand, the relatively intimate union between shoe and foot is lost when an internal shoe is interposed, and additional alterations to the retail shoe are almost invariably required.

According to REGENSPURGER (1975), the prescription of an internal shoe is indicated in:

1. Leg inequality
2. Forefoot loss
3. Flaccid and spastic paralysis
4. Major foot deformity.

To a certain extent, therefore, internal shoes may function as limb-lengthening orthoses, as partial foot prostheses or as internal shoes for paralysis.

3.8.1 Internal Shoe for Leg Inequality (Limb-Lengthening Orthosis)

In moderate leg inequality (approximately 7 to 12 cm or 2.8 to 4.8 inches) an orthopedic shoe plus an internal shoe is recommended; in the event of greater inequality, an O'Connor boot should be used.

In the former case the internal shoe is made of casting resin or hard foam material. It should lace up at the front and extend forward as far as the metatarsophalangeal joints (see Fig. 51). To ensure that it fits well inside the cladding shoe (outer shoe) and is not too obvious, the foot should be supported in equinus.

The *O'Connor boot* is a type of orthopedic appliance in which the internal shoe is positioned either at right angles to the lower leg or in equinus inside a leather casing fashioned like a shoe upper (see Fig. 52). As with a prosthesis, an artificial foot is then positioned below the internal shoe and fitted with a retail shoe. The insole shape of the artificial foot and its heel pitch should therefore be adjusted to match the retail shoe.

In female patients it is sometimes advisable on cosmetic grounds to bring the foot of the very much shorter leg into extreme equinus, if necessary even by surgical means, and then to build a type of orthosis into which the foot and lower leg enter from behind.

3.8.2 Internal Shoe for Forefoot Loss

As a general rule, metatarsal stumps should be catered for with an orthopedic shoe whereas tarsal stumps require an internal shoe. However, several exceptions to this rule are permitted. For example, it is very probable that metatarsal stumps in female patients could also be compensated using an internal shoe.

The internal shoe for forefoot loss incorporates the following orthopedic elements:

1. *Forefoot filler:* this may be made of a variety of materials and replaces the lost foot section inside the shoe (see Fig. 61). It resembles the toe part of the universally familiar shoe-tree. The forefoot filler does not merely serve to fill out space inside the orthopedic shoe, but may also include additional elements, such as pressure-loaded springs (Schlüter forefoot prosthesis, Fig. 61), a stiffened tongue (Welsch internal shoe prosthesis, Fig. 62), or an anterior tibial plate which serves to transmit force (Teufel forefoot prosthesis, Fig. 63).

2. An *(anterior) moulded leather stiffener* is also required; this may be of varying stiffness and serves to transmit gravity from the tibia to the forefoot filler. The greater the forefoot area to be replaced, the higher and stiffer the element required. In Pirogoff's amputation, the stiffener is a foam-cushioned, Ortholene tibial plate (referred to by Marquardt as a "knemide" from the Greek word κνημίς meaning "shin pad"). Moreover, the stiffener is best attached to the forefoot filler rather than to the insole.

A metatarsal bar is indispensable here and care should always be taken to ensure that it is positioned correctly proximal to the end of the stump in order to counteract the equinus tendency of the stump at all times.

The heel counter of the internal shoe should fit snugly against the calcaneus, ensuring a firm grip and preventing increased movement. The calcaneus should be deeply supported: the shorter the stump, the deeper the support. More precise details may be found in section 5.6.

3.8.3 Internal Shoe for Paralysis

3.8.3.1 Flaccid Paralysis

In this context, especially in the management of peroneal nerve paralysis, internal shoes are advantageous in that they are relatively unobtrusive. They consist of a strong footplate combined with a stiffener which extends proximally behind the calcaneus. In addition, the dorsiflexing effect can be increased using rubber traction elements which extend from the lower leg to the forefoot.

The *Kraus internal shoe for flaccid paralysis* also includes an upper which extends beyond the metatarsophalangeal joints (see Fig. 55). The stiffener forks medially and laterally above the malleoli so as not to exert pressure on the Achilles tendon.

3.8.3.2 Spastic Paralysis

An internal shoe may possibly be indicated in adults with spastic paralysis. If equinus does not increase on ground contact, and provided no further damage is caused, correction may be attempted using the principles outlined for the paralytic equinus foot. Otherwise, the equinus foot has to be fully compensated, in which case an internal shoe is not appropriate (see also 5.2.5).

3.8.4 Internal Shoe for Major Foot Deformity

In certain circumstances severe toe and foot deformities can be catered for more effectively with an internal shoe than with an orthopedic shoe alone, particularly in cases where pressure on painful scars or exostoses has to be relieved, and friction between foot and footwear has to be kept to an absolute minimum. It is a simple matter to recess and line these points on the internal shoe.

4 The Perpendicular Construction of the Orthopedic Shoe

In order to understand what is meant by the perpendicular construction of the shoe, it will probably be helpful to begin by explaining a few concepts.

Two forces act on the foot during standing: *one half of the bodyweight acts downwards from the centre of gravity* while an equal but opposite force, the *ground reactive force,* is applied to the foot by the floor. In a person standing

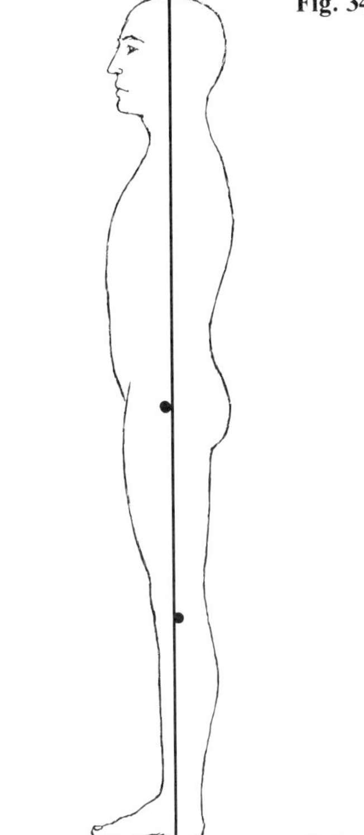

Fig. 34. Gravity line during erect stance

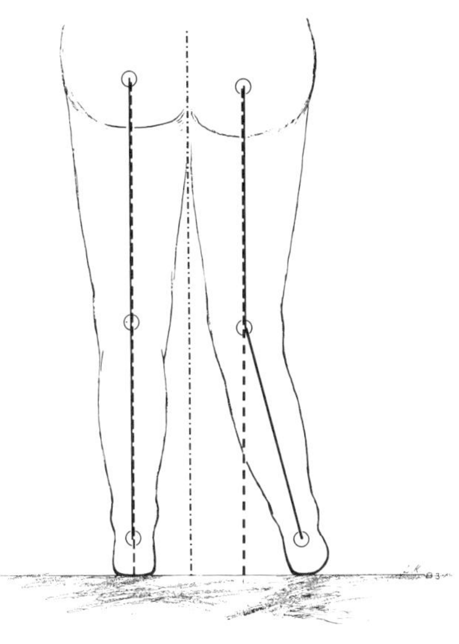

Fig. 35. Weight line and perpendicular. Left normal; right in genu valgum

erect with legs straight and slightly apart, the resultant line of these forces passes through the midpoint of the hip joint via the midpoint of the knee and ankle joints to a point on the ground slightly in front of the heel strike surface (Fig. 34). With the knee joint flexed but with body position otherwise unchanged, this force line would pass behind the knee joint and exert a bending force on it.

In orthopedic shoe technology, the gravity line is also known as the *perpendicular,* and should be distinguished from the *weight line.* In simple terms, the weight line is the line along which material force is transmitted in reality. In a normal individual standing perfectly erect, the weight line follows the same course as the perpendicular from the midpoint of the hip joint through the midpoint of the ankle joint to the talus (Fig. 35). Thereafter, however, it divides into two lines, one of which extends forward to the tip of the second toe (in fact, two lines extend forward: one to the first metatarsal head and the other to the fifth metatarsal head), while the other extends down to the apex of the plantar surface of the calcaneus. The resultant of the ground reactive force also follows this weight line, but is of course applied in the opposite direction (Fig. 36).

When the knee joint is flexed, the perpendicular and the weight line no longer coincide in the thigh and lower leg. The weight line continues to follow the anatomical line of the leg, but now has an additional bend at the knee joint. The same situation obtains in genu valgum and genu varum, although in these circumstances the weight line is bent and deviates from the perpendicular in the frontal rather than in the sagittal plane (Fig. 35).

When the weight line and the perpendicular in erect stance no longer coincide in the thigh and lower leg, as in genu valgum and genu varum, the force of gravity acts as a lever to exacerbate the existing deformity. The greater the deviation between the two lines, the more pronounced this exacerbation.

In the context of perpendicular shoe construction it is thus critically important to define the normal weight-bearing surface, i.e. the normal stand of the shoe, such as would be measured in an individual with healthy legs. This should be regarded as axiomatic and an unchanging goal, regardless of the deformity present. Consequently, where a deformity does exist, the shoemaker should proceed as if it did not exist at all, always provided that perpendicular construction is really desired and it is not necessary to forsake its principles for any particular reason. Formulated as a shoe construction goal, this rule might then read as follows: *Even in the diseased foot, the weight line should be applied to the weight-bearing surface of the shoe as it would be in a normal individual.* However, this means that the normal theoretical weight-bearing surface of the shoe needs to be determined in each case.

The perpendicular is of vital importance in *determining the weight-bearing surface of the shoe* as it would be in a healthy individual because, in normal erect stance, it coincides with the weight line as far as the talus. However, since

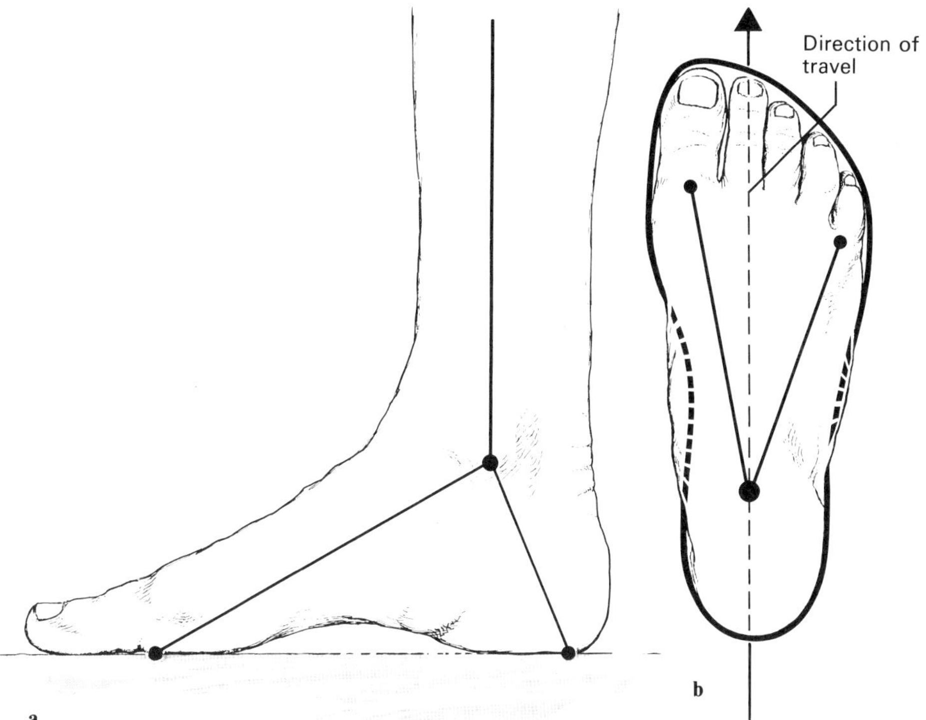

Fig. 36a, b. Weight lines in the foot. **a** Medial view. **b** From above showing weight-bearing surface

it is impossible to determine the perpendicular from the midpoint of the hip joint, two makeshift lines (the posterior and lateral perpendiculars) are used, irrespective of whether an orthopedic shoe, an internal shoe or a prosthesis to correct leg inequality is to be constructed. In establishing the basis for perpendicular shoe construction (synonymous with determining the weight-bearing surface of a hypothetical normal leg or, more accurately, foot), reference is made to *sagittal and frontal perpendicular construction.*

In practice, the *posterior perpendicular* is measured using the line dropped from the midpoint of the buttock (Fig. 37). The point projected to the ground with the plumb line is then marked on a base plate. The *lateral perpendicular* is measured from the greater trochanter and the point projected for it is also marked. The weight-bearing surface of the shoe is then found by drawing a straight line forward in the direction of travel from the point projected for the posterior perpendicular. A second line is then drawn from the point projected for the lateral perpendicular to join the first line at right angles. The first line extends to the tip of the second toe, and the line drawn at right angles to it (passing through the lateral projection point) marks the front edge of the shoe heel (heel breast) of the hypothetical normal shoe.

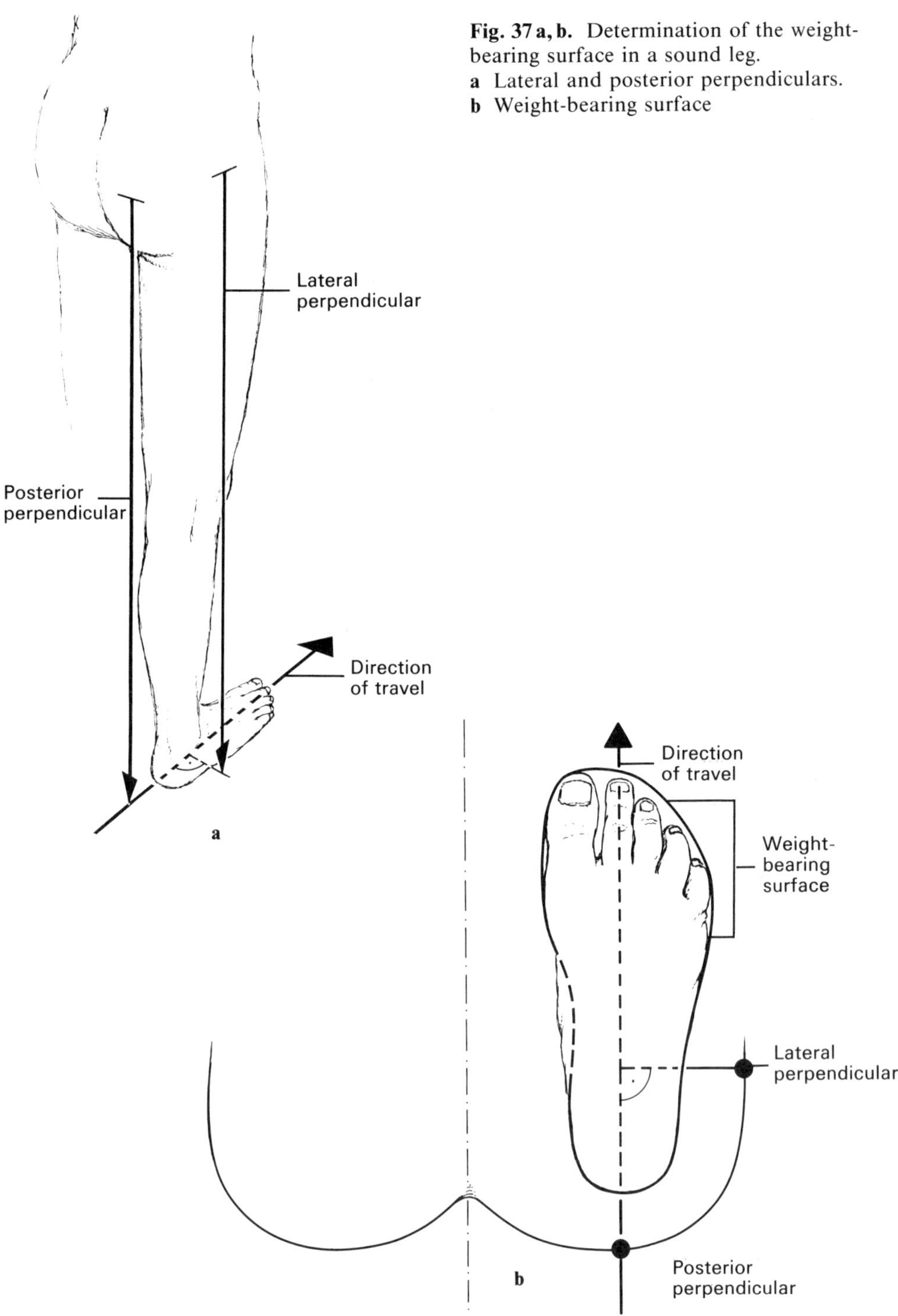

Fig. 37 a, b. Determination of the weight-bearing surface in a sound leg.
a Lateral and posterior perpendiculars.
b Weight-bearing surface

In the perpendicular construction of an orthopedic shoe, therefore, the front edge of the shoe heel also coincides with the straight line drawn at right angles to the direction of travel, and the tip of the second toe is also visualised as lying on the longitudinal straight line. This applies whatever the foot deformity. The shoe bottom (usually a cork-like material) is then positioned perpendicularly as a foundation between the deformed foot and the weight-bearing surface of the shoe (shoe sole) so that the placement of the outsole is determined not by the deformed foot but by the leg.

The actions of pathological forces due to deformity can be reduced only by perpendicular shoe construction which relieves pressure and facilitates roll-over.

The reduction of deforming forces will now be illustrated taking genu valgum as an example (Fig. 38). In this condition, the weight line deviates from the perpendicular in the frontal plane. The point projected for the perpendicular deviates medially from the point at which the ground reactive force acts on the calcaneus. The distance between these two points on the ground is proportional to the valgus leverage acting on the knee joint during standing. Medial repositioning of the shoe bottom (and hence of the weight-bearing surface of the shoe) brings the point of application of the ground reactive force closer to the point projected for the perpendicular, thus reducing the leverage responsible for the valgus deformity. Exactly the same procedure would be adopted in pes valgus. In this case, too, the weight line deviates laterally from the perpendicular, and medial displacement of the shoe bottom will reduce the valgus forces in the subtalar joint.

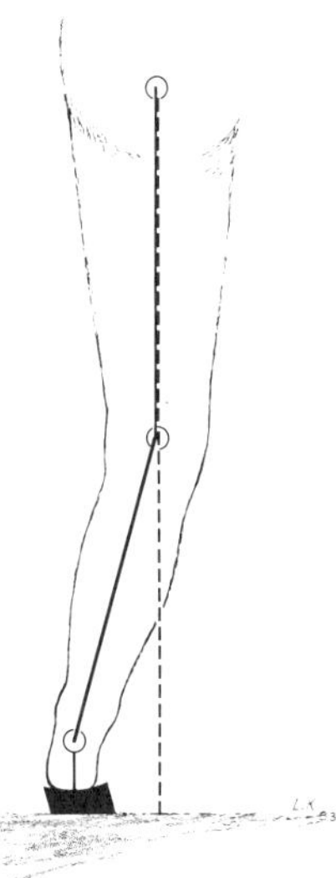

Fig. 38. Perpendicular construction in genu valgum with pes valgus (from Regenspurger)

Perpendicular construction becomes complicated in the presence of two coexisting deformities which should ideally be treated by moving the weight-bearing surface in opposite directions, e.g. varus deformity at the knee joint and valgus deformity in the subtalar joint. In this particular example, if genu varum is corrected by perpendicular shoe construction, the valgus forces acting on the subtalar joint become even greater. In such cases, both deformities cannot be corrected simultaneously. It is then necessary in each individual case to decide which deformity is the more disabling, severe or painful in standing and moving and to correct that one only. As a rule this will probably be the deformity which exerts the greater mechanical effect as a result of the longer lever involved. In the management of genu varum accompanied by pes valgus, for example, the tendency would be to treat genu varum by moving the shoe bottom laterally while leaving pes valgus uncorrected.

As demonstrated in the example of genu valgum, *perpendicular shoe construction* also *relieves* sections of joint or bone under pathologically elevated pressure; in genu valgum, for example, it relieves pressure on the lateral part of the knee joint. The same also applies to the foot. In clubfoot, for example, perpendicular construction reduces supinating forces to some extent and simultaneously relieves pressure. The principles of perpendicular construction are also *important for rollover.* Perpendicular construction simulates normal conditions in that the sagittal (longitudinal) axis of the weight-bearing surface extends to the tip of the second toe. Consequently, the resultant of the body's gravitational force moves continuously along the components of the weight line in the foot from the calcaneus via the metatarsus to the tip of the second toe. However, if the principles of perpendicular construction are ignored, forces result which lie outside the weight-bearing surface, uncomfortable pressure is exerted on the foot due to the wrongly constructed shoe, and there may be a tendency for the foot to slip out of the shoe.

5 Indications for Orthopedic Footwear and Prescription Examples

The clearest and most comprehensive definition of the orthopedic shoe was in fact given in 1953 by the Advisory Committee of the German Orthopedic Society. "The orthopedic shoe is a therapeutic aid employed by the orthopedic specialist. It is custom-made for the individual diseased or deformed foot using special techniques of measurement and design. As well as shodding the foot, it provides individualised requisite features such as padding, pressure relief, support, defect compensation or correction, and aids to immobilisation or heel-to-toe movement. 'Orthopedic shoes' which are mass-produced or made on a series last are not worthy of the name, even though they may take account of individual features of the deformity."

The two signal characteristics of the orthopedic shoe are therefore that it must be custom-made for one individual foot and that it is a medical, therapeutic aid. Both criteria serve to distinguish it from the retail shoe which is factory-produced on a mass scale and is not intended to fit one specific foot to the exclusion of all others.

Orthopedic elements may also be added subsequently to a retail shoe, for example, a rocker bar in hallux rigidus. Such measures are always suitable for patients for whom management using a custom-made shoe would not only be disproportionately expensive but would also be excessively prodigal of effort and time. While the prescription of an orthopedic element is the responsibility of the medical profession and the element itself is an aid to medical treatment, this does not make the retail shoe an orthopedic shoe. These elements added to production-line retail footwear are known as *modifications to the retail shoe.*

In this chapter, which focuses attention on the orthopedic disorders for treatment, the indications for the orthopedic shoe and for modifications to retail footwear are usually stated explicitly, but are not dealt with separately in special sections. The inserts most commonly employed are also dealt with in this chapter since it would be incomplete to omit all reference to them in connection with orthopedic footwear.

The orthopedic shoe is occasionally nothing more than a compromise solution, and even then, not always the best. This is true in two senses. Firstly, many disorders might well be treated differently (and sometimes more effectively) in other ways, for example, by surgery or with an orthotic device (orthopedic appliance). Secondly, the orthopedic element described here may not always completely achieve in functional terms what it appears to promise in theory. In such cases the physico-mechanical characteristics of the element are simply insufficient to replace natural function totally. This lies in the mechanical nature of the element which is intended merely as a substitute.

Like any other medical remedy, the orthopedic shoe must have an *adequate prescription*. A poorly written prescription is the clearest indicator of defective detailed knowledge of the potential individual functions of the orthopedic shoe. To date there are no detailed absolute guidelines governing the prescription of orthopedic footwear. This applies both with regard to indications and to actual prescription writing. An orthopedic shoe is indicated whenever it is anticipated that it will considerably improve standing or walking ability and whenever surgery has been refused, is contra-indicated for specific reasons or would merely achieve the same result incompletely if at all.

A reasonably complete prescription should take account of the following particulars:

1. The type of footwear.
2. The method of construction (plaster cast or made-to-measure).
3. The design of the upper.
4. The need for compensatory support.
5. The design of the insole in cases where compensatory support is not necessary.
6. The design of the outsole.
7. The height of the heel and, where appropriate, whether a buffer heel is indicated.
8. Possibly, the type of leather from which the upper is to be made.
9. The diagnosis (absolutely essential).

Of course, the above points need not be listed individually on the prescription. *The essential characteristic of a complete prescription is that the shoemaker should know which orthopedic elements the shoe requires.*

A few additional remarks on the prescription examples given in this chapter will be helpful. Unlike medicines and like units of weight, the orthopedic shoe should be referred to in the accusative case on the prescription. There is also no objection to the frequent use of arabic numerals for clarity or ease of understanding. However, in correct prescription writing, it is improper to use the numeral 1 for "a" or "an": strictly speaking, it should only be used to indicate "one".

It has not always been explicitly stated that orthopedic elements, e.g. orthopedic bars or compensation for a short leg, may sometimes be required on the sound foot as a result of measures implemented on the deformed foot.

For the sake of uniformity, the left foot or leg has always been taken to be defective/deformed in the prescription examples in this chapter.

For some readers, several of the prescriptions proposed in these pages may be redundant or, at the very least, some statements in them may be superfluous. For example, the rigid rocker-sole shoe is such a precisely defined entity that it probably does not require further explanation. On the other hand, experienced practitioners may regret the occasional total omission of express reference to a particular orthopedic element. Prescriptions for orthopedic footwear are not standardised, and this permits considerable individual latitude in prescription writing. It is self-evident that prescriptions need to be appropriate for the individual case in question. Those presented here are intended primarily to stimulate the reader to remember the most important orthopedic elements and to convey an idea of the shoe as a whole.

5.1 Foot and Toe Deformities

5.1.1 Pes Cavus

Simple pes cavus is characterised by only one deformity in a single plane, the sagittal plane. Frequently, however, the condition is accompanied by claw toes and splayfoot or a dorsal prominence.

It is incorrect procedure in pes cavus to position the longitudinal arch on an insert or compensatory support in the normal way because this will lift the

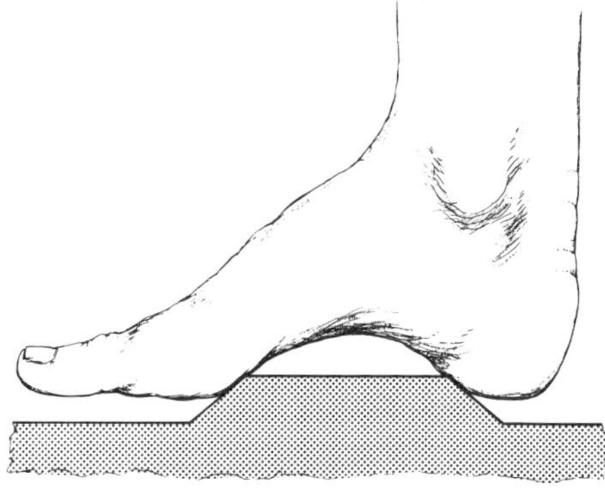

Fig. 39. Low cavus insole

plantar aponeurosis even higher and the heel will move even closer to the metatarsal heads. This would merely aggravate pes cavus.

The correct procedure is to use a *low cavus insole* (Fig. 39) which causes flattening of the longitudinal arch over two angled planes, one of which lies behind the metatarsal heads while the other is positioned in front of the apex of the plantar surface of the calcaneus. Where splayfoot is also present, the low cavus insole may also be fitted with a metatarsal pad. Rollover may be encouraged by a rocker bar placed slightly further back than usual; however, this should not be too high because it might lead to gait unsteadiness by further reducing the weight-bearing surface of the sole.

If the condition is not too extreme and does not present as pes equinoexcavatus, pes cavus in children should not be treated with shoes, but simply with an insert incorporating a low cavus insole. In adults it is generally sufficient either to modify the retail shoes or to use a metal insert incorporating a corrective low cavus insole and a metatarsal pad, where appropriate. The insert should also have a medial anterior and posterior flange and a lateral flange. Lateral stiffening of the shoe bottom will counteract the common tendency to supination and can also be prescribed as a modification.

The prescription for modifications to retail shoes should read as for the inserts. *Orthopedic shoes are only appropriate if the deformity threatens to develop in a second plane and if there has been contracture in some joints*, thus impairing rollover.

> Rx: One pair of low orthopedic shoes, made-to-measure, with low cavus insole, concealed rocker bar placed slightly further back than usual, with reinforced heel counter and buffer heel. Lateral stiffening of the shoe bottom.
> Diagnosis: Partially contracted pes cavus.

If the foot is not balanced to the ground, the sole and heel of the shoe should be displaced laterally in line with the principles of perpendicular construction. Special care should be taken to ensure that the shoe is long enough.

5.1.2 Pes Equinoexcavatus

The conservative management of pes equinoexcavatus is much more problematic and is essentially inadequate. Pes equinoexcavatus differs fundamentally from pes cavus not merely in terms of aetiology: it is characterised by deformity in more than one plane and is generally of a progressive nature. There is usually an underlying neurological disorder, the progressive course of which includes the foot deformity. Pes equinoexcavatus may also be associated with increased forefoot pronation, claw toes and splayfoot. The foot in Friedreich's ataxia is further characterised by equinus. Although patients with this condition are sometimes only able to walk again in orthopedic footwear, corrective surgery remains the treatment of choice for pes equinoexcavatus and for clubfoot. Despite this fact, the principles of footwear provision will be delineated here. For once, however, no prescription will be offered because this needs to be adapted to the individual patient and is relatively straightforward to deduce. A prescription example here might all too easily deflect the reader into thinking along conservative lines instead of giving the surgical approach due priority.

A low cavus insole can have little point here because it is virtually impossible to flatten the longitudinal arch. A *stepped insole* would thus appear to make rather more sense provided that it is also constructed as a support. A metatarsal pad should only be incorporated if relatively severe equinus is absent.

Caution should be exercised with the fitting of orthopedic bars because these reduce gait stability. The upper should be *reinforced with heel counters*. The first ray should not be deeply padded, but the third and fourth metatarsal heads should be raised (Rabl's recommendation). The lateral shoe bottom should be stiffened. In functional terms, this may be achieved most efficiently by fitting a lateral sole wedge which also has the effect of compensating for leg inequality. A *buffer heel* will counteract pain in the region of the calcaneus.

If the foot is not balanced to the ground, the heel and sole of the shoe should be displaced laterally. The toe space should be enlarged to provide increased accommodation for claw toes. Ideally, the plantar surface of the joint line should be cushioned and finally, in pes equinoexcavatus in particular, the shoe should be sufficiently long.

5.1.3 Talipes Calcaneus

Because they are managed in different ways, contracted talipes calcaneus and passively correctable pes calcaneoexcavatus due to paralysis will be dealt with separately.

5.1.3.1 Contracted Talipes Calcaneus

In this condition the provision of orthopedic footwear is simply an emergency solution in cases where surgery is not possible or has been refused. In such circumstances, a *rocker-sole shoe* should be prescribed comprising the following four elements: metatarsal bar, round-edge heel, wedge heel and a non-slip sole. Because of the increased risk of slippage, an extended heel is recommended in place of the wedge heel. However, the main disadvantage of the rocker-sole shoe in this condition is that the forefoot has to be raised relatively high, thus impairing rollover and lending the shoe a generally clumsy appearance. The calcaneus should be deeply padded and the shoe should carry a flat heel.

Rx: One pair of orthopedic shoes with rocker-sole shoe left (plaster cast), with compensatory support which raises the line of the metatarsal heads, a metatarsal bar and deep padding for the calcaneus. Round-edge heel extended forward.
Diagnosis: Contracted talipes calcaneus left.

5.1.3.2 Pes Calcaneoexcavatus due to Paralysis

Rabl is certainly correct when writing of the management of this deformity: "The chances of affording relief without recourse to surgery are by no means as poor as many orthopedic specialists believe." However, as RABL (1982) also notes, this depends "on the avoidance of one besetting error. The shoe in tibial nerve paralysis should not be made as an ankle boot, but as a *low shoe*".

Since this deformity is caused by paralysis of the tibial nerve, the sole of the foot also has diminished contact sensitivity. Consequently, extra care is required to ensure that the foot enjoys elastic support without localised pressure points, otherwise there is a danger that pressure sores may develop.

The provision of footwear in the management of this condition should seek to lengthen the posterior lever arm to facilitate plantar flexion, to press the cal-

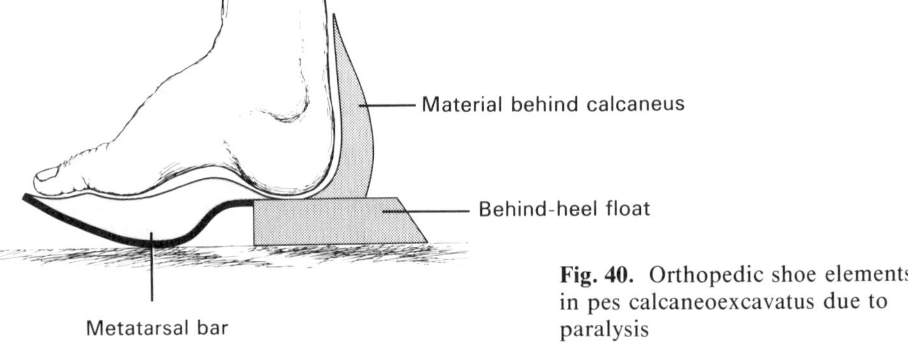

Fig. 40. Orthopedic shoe elements in pes calcaneoexcavatus due to paralysis

caneus up and back if possible, and to shorten the anterior lever arm. A behind-heel float will encourage plantar flexion. Some degree of calcaneal correction can be achieved using a stepped insole, although care should be taken to ensure that there is sufficient space inside the shoe behind the heel to enable the calcaneus to be levered far enough up and back by the ground reactive force. A felt pad 2 to 3 cm (0.8 to 1.2 inches) thick placed behind the heel will give this degree of latitude and also offers the advantage of lengthening the posterior lever arm. The metatarsal bar shortens the anterior lever arm (Fig. 40).

Rx: One pair of low orthopedic shoes, plaster cast, with behind-heel float left, felt pad 2.5 cm (1 inch) thick behind left heel and compensatory support left with a relatively high metatarsal bar, a corrective step in front of the calcaneus and elastic support for the remainder of the plantar surface of the foot.

Diagnosis: Pes calcaneoexcavatus due to paralysis left.

5.1.4 Clubfoot

This is not the place to enlarge upon the view that a clubfoot which requires an orthopedic shoe has been inappropriately treated. It simply has to be accepted that clubfoot may require such management, rare though this may be in civilised countries. However, anyone who has been called upon to treat patients from parts of the world where the modern techniques of clubfoot management are not yet normative will be only too familiar with this distressing fact.

Nevertheless, while clubfoot is of major significance in orthopedic practice, inordinate attention should not be devoted here to the provision of orthopedic footwear, firstly because this is and should remain a genuinely rare solution and secondly because orthopedic practitioners should not be misled into thinking too readily along these lines. For this reason, the principles of shoe management will be presented more as general rules for practice, however appealing it might seem to use the clubfoot condition to re-emphasise certain rules of shoe mechanics (e.g. perpendicular construction). The reader who is more interested in the theoretical aspects should consult the specialist literature, in particular the work of Marquardt.

Firstly, according to Marquardt, it is essential to draw the following distinctions:

1. Between stable and collapsed clubfoot. In stable clubfoot (provided contracture is absent), the ground reactive force may still correct supination. The essential mechanical precondition here is that the posterior perpendicular

dropped from the hip joint should pass medially by the base and head of the fifth metatarsal. However, if the perpendicular is lateral to this point (collapsed clubfoot), the ground reactive force will aggravate supination and cause the clubfoot to "collapse" even further.

2. Between clubfoot which is still amenable to passive correction and contracted clubfoot. In the former case, inserts or shoes can still exert varying degrees of correction on the three clubfoot components. In contracted clubfoot, however, even to attempt such correction would be incorrect and harmful.

The first principle of correction is embodied in the *three-point system (Fig.* 41) in which two forces are applied in one direction, while a third force is applied centrally in the opposite direction to counteract the deformity, in this case adduction of the foot. The second principle is to exploit the *ground reactive force* (directed against supination and equinus). In the three-point system, one force is applied to the medial aspect of the calcaneus while a second similarly directed force is applied behind the first metatarsal head; the third and opposite central force is applied to the lateral border of the foot at the level of the cuboid bone. The ground reactive force to discourage supination tendencies should also act on the cuboid bone and this can be achieved most effectively using a Berlakovits stepped insole in which the front step should be positioned immediately behind the fifth metatarsal head (see also 3.2.2). A lateral flare on the shoe bottom and heel will also serve to counteract supination. Deep positioning of the calcaneus and a flat heel are useful in correcting equinus.

The principal characteristics of *contracted clubfoot* are overload discomfort and diminished rollover. The lateral border of the foot, and the fifth metatarsal head in particular, are the main points under pressure. The stepped insole, used here in an identical fashion to relieve pressure, alleviates pain most effi-

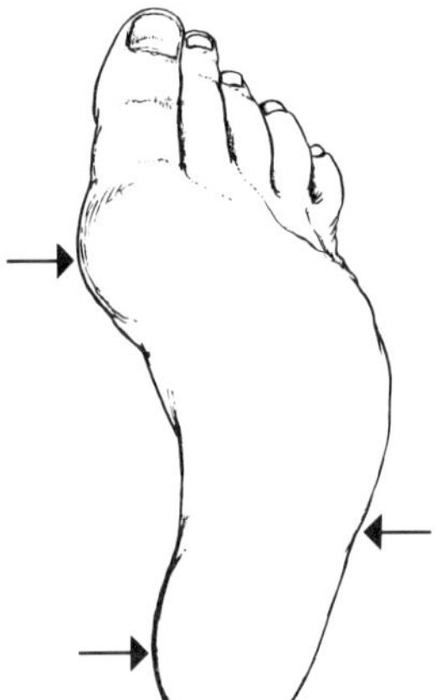

Fig. 41. Three-point system for the correction of the adduction component in clubfoot

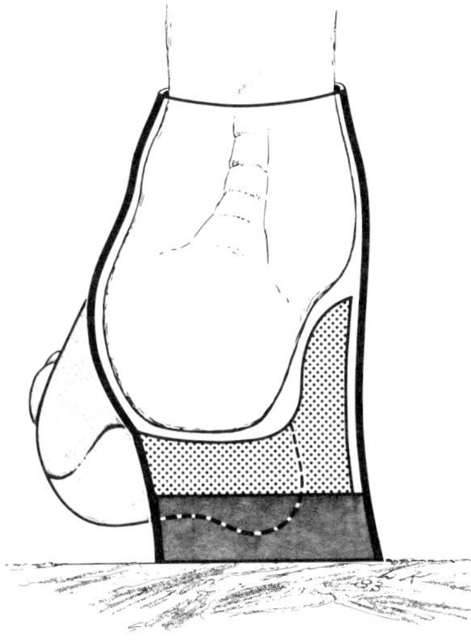

Fig. 42. Perpendicular construction for clubfoot which is still amenable to passive correction. The shoe heel and support are displaced laterally

ciently in clubfoot which is still stable. Bony prominences should be padded more generously, as appropriate, and a metatarsal bar is very often beneficial.

In the *collapsed, contracted clubfoot* management is particularly problematic if the forefoot still points forward. In such circumstances, in order to relieve the lateral border of the foot, a recess may be made in the support in such a way that the fifth metatarsal head is under less pressure.

The shoe bottom in this case should be flat and angular (MARQUARDT, 1965). Its lateral border should not be too thick because this is worn down especially easily and the pronating effect is lost (REGENSPURGER, 1975). If fitted at all, any orthopedic bar should be of only miniscule thickness.

Adherence to the rules of perpendicular shoe construction is of absolute importance in clubfoot in particular. In the foot which is still susceptible to passive correction, the shoe heel and support should be displaced laterally (Fig. 42). The last must be kept straight so as to make the stand of the shoe coincide as closely as possible with the weight-bearing surface during rollover.

It is quite wrong to prescribe shoes for correctable clubfoot in children because the shoe cannot possibly fit the growing foot and will soon forfeit any corrective effect. A metal insert is the remedy of choice in such cases, especially where surgery has been performed and there is a risk of relapse.

Rx: One pair of made-to-measure metal inserts (or plaster cast if the deformity is too extreme) with strong support for the left cuboid bone, with a well-fitting lateral flange, a medial flange at the left calcaneus, an elongated lateral flange at the great toe and with the heel supported in mild calcaneus.

Diagnosis: Corrected clubfoot in infancy.

Rx: One pair of laced orthopedic ankle boots (plaster cast) with stable heel counter left extending laterally as far as the cuboid bone and medially as far as the first metatarsal head; compensatory support with a step underneath the cuboid bone and behind the fifth metatarsal head left, stiffened laterally and with the calcaneus supported rather more deeply. Eisenmann strap. Shoe bottom and flat lateral Thomas heel displaced laterally in accordance with perpendicular construction principles.
Diagnosis: Corrected stable clubfoot left.

Rx: One pair of laced ankle boots (or low shoes in milder cases), plaster cast, with compensatory support left, with a step underneath the cuboid bone and behind the fifth metatarsal head, with cushioned recesses for painful prominences and a metatarsal bar 0.5 cm (0.2 inches) high. Shoe bottom and lateral Thomas heel displaced laterally. Soft soles.
Diagnosis: Contracted clubfoot left.

Management of the overturned foot is extremely difficult. In completely over-turned and adducted feet, it is best to prescribe an O'Connor boot which will support the foot properly and firmly, but which takes no account of the deformity (see Fig. 52). The support padding of the O'Connor boot should of course be as deep as possible.

Rx: One pair of orthopedic shoes (plaster cast), with O'Connor boot left, with elastic support padding and internal fastening, and with cushioned recesses for prominent tender areas; perpendicular construction of the internal shoe and the retail shoe. Metatarsal bar right.
Diagnosis: Extremely deformed clubfoot left.

5.1.5 Pes Adductus (Sickle Foot)

In our opinion this foot deformity should never be considered as a true candidate for orthopedic footwear. In fact, even inserts are only indicated with reservation and in full awareness of the exceptional circumstances. There are three reasons for this:

1. Surgery is the proper treatment for severe pes adductus which cannot be compensated.

2. The correction of this anomaly would have to be in line with the three-point system (see Fig. 41). The posterior force would then be applied medial to the calcaneus, thus accentuating the already valgus heel.

3. If any corrective measures at all are used, then a metal insert should be sufficient. Prescription of an orthopedic shoe would be tantamount to overtreatment, quite apart from the fact that pes adductus (provided it is only mild) causes hardly any discomfort.

5.1.6 Pes Planovalgus (Pes Planotransversus)

In therapeutic terms it is of cardinal importance to differentiate between actively correctable and passively correctable planotransversus foot and the contracted planovalgus foot.

If the longitudinal arch is raised and the calcaneus goes into varus when a child stands on tiptoe, it is legitimate to speak of an *actively correctable planotransversus foot*. Quite simply and concisely, the actively correctable planotransversus foot should only be treated with active exercises (physiotherapy) and with properly fitting footwear (see 1.3).

Treatment of the *passively correctable planotransversus foot* should be active and passive simultaneously, whereas support and relief of pressure are the principal goals in the *passively contracted planovalgus foot*. Consequently, the planotransversus foot which can be actively raised is not a candidate for orthopedic footwear (except possibly for a supination wedge).

5.1.6.1 Passively Correctable Planotransversus Foot

Here, too, the principles governing the active strengthening of the foot should not be underestimated or ignored: foot gymnastics and walking barefoot are especially important.

Modifications to retail shoes are normally sufficient in cases where the planotransversus foot can still be actively raised to a certain extent. The older orthopedic school realised one fact which is still important today: the planotransversus foot should be corrected from the hindfoot, i. e. heel pronation should be discouraged. In the first instance this may be achieved using a *supination wedge* (see 3.7.5). The typical planotransversus foot is out of torsion, i. e. the hindfoot is pronated and the forefoot is supinated. The supination wedge supinates the hindfoot again to a major extent and thus creates the conditions for physiological torsion. Wherever possible, the attempt should be made to manage with the supination wedge alone. Care should be taken here to ensure that the crown of the curvature of the wedge is located accurately, i. e. at the point where the perpendicular dropped from the tip of the medial malleolus intersects the ground plane. If the retail shoe does not have a flexible waist, the effect of the supination wedge can be increased by using a medially elongated heel (medial Thomas heel).

If the hindfoot remains pronated despite this measure, its position can be counteracted by using a *heel which is displaced and flared medially*.

If prescribed, inserts should be constructed in accordance with the principles outlined earlier. Wherever possible, the heel cup alone should suffice. In this case, the support under the sustentaculum tali corresponds to the supination wedge. The heel cup should fit exactly to the hindfoot so as not to slip about and, to be fully effective, it requires a highly flexible shoe. Two critical points should be noted here.

Firstly, inserts should never be automatically prescribed for planotransversus feet: even though it may not be totally correctable, not every planotransversus foot necessarily requires an insert. This applies especially for the non-painful planotransversus foot whose function remains undisturbed.

Secondly, some otherwise excellent specialist textbooks in this field still insist that a raised heel can counteract footdrop because it straightens the calcaneus and relieves the foot of some elements of heel-to-toe movement. This is clearly not correct. A raised heel would only reduce muscle activity and increase the load on the ball of the foot. In particular, it is important that the valgus position of the hindfoot should, without exception, be corrected actively, rather than passively by a raised heel which would only be disadvantageous.

The corrective planotransversus foot insert (made of metal, leather-lined cork or plastic) performs both a supportive and a corrective function. It supports the sustentaculum tali and extends only as far as the plantar surface beneath the first metatarsal head, so as to exert torsion on the forefoot as well. Apart from an admittedly slight pronating effect on the forefoot, this insert offers no major advantages over the supination wedge.

The *Hohmann torsion insert* is reserved for use in planotransversus feet which can be raised passively only with great difficulty and in which forefoot supination is relatively more pronounced. As a rule the Hohmann insert is made of metal and its anterior edge extends laterally beyond the fourth and fifth metatarsophalangeal joints, in order to exert even more marked torsion on the foot (see Fig. 43).

With this particular insert there is a recess for the plantar surface beneath the great toe. The Hohmann insert has one disadvantage: it requires laced ankle boots or low shoes with a high top line because the hindfoot can easily be levered out of the shoe during walking.

The *Volkmann winged torsion insert* (named after a Ravensburg orthopedic specialist and not the surgeon from Halle) is also intended for use in the planotransversus foot which can be raised passively only with difficulty (Fig. 44). Its

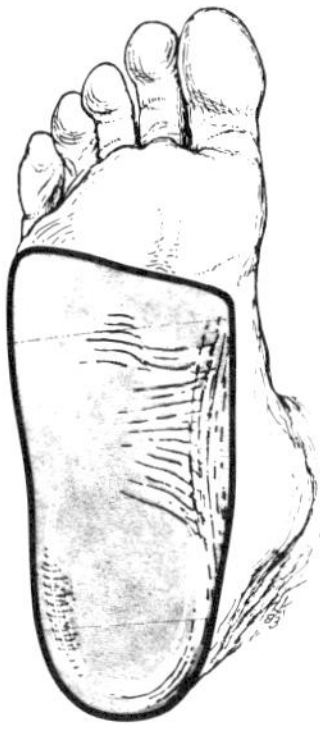

Fig. 43. Hohmann torsion insert

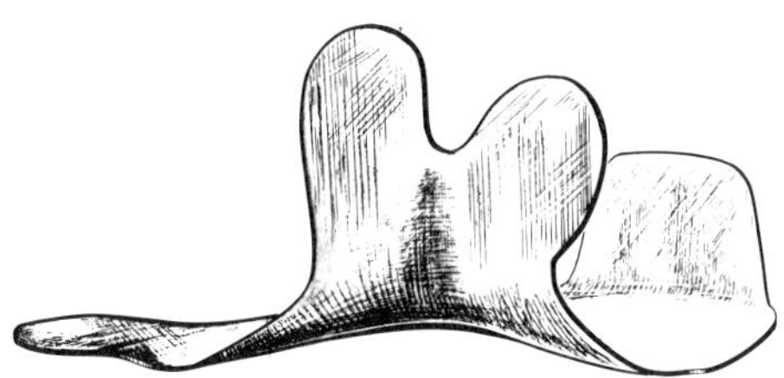

Fig. 44. Volkmann winged torsion insert

underlying principle is to keep the hindfoot supinated by means of winged flanges positioned medially and laterally. The medial flange is heart-shaped; its proximal lobe grips the calcaneus and its distal lobe grips the navicular bone. The metal sole extends forward like a narrow bridge to behind the second to fourth metatarsal heads and is itself torqued in such a way that during load bearing, it raises the longitudinal arch of the foot.

These shoe modifications are simple to prescribe once the requisite measurements have been taken. When supplying inserts, it is sufficient to write either:

Rx: One pair of Hohmann torsion inserts, metal, made to measure or
Rx: One pair of Volkmann winged torsion inserts, metal, made to measure.
Diagnosis: Passively correctable planotransversus foot.

Orthopedic shoes are really not indicated for passively correctable planotransversus feet and would probably constitute a form of overtreatment.

5.1.6.2 Contracted Planovalgus Foot

Active therapy plays only a minor role in this deformity and is used primarily to strengthen muscles which are becoming atrophied as a result of pressure-relieving and supportive measures. In this context, use of the Thomsen foot gymnastic slipperette for several hours at a time is to be recommended.

Firstly, it is important to note that the contracted planovalgus foot should not be confused with the inflamed contracted valgus foot. The former clinical condition is due not to valgus foot as such, but to the process of becoming flatfooted, i.e. it is a dynamic rather than a static condition. Accordingly, discomfort is often experienced acutely. Almost invariably, standing on the medial or lateral border of the foot suddenly becomes impossible due to pain and the onset of contracture, and pain is generally also perceived across the entire tarsal and metatarsal regions.

In the valgus foot which is merely contracted, discomfort is a rather less prominent feature. However, it is typical that heel pronation and forefoot supination cannot even be corrected passively. The gait is awkward, and because the anterior lever of the foot is longer due to flattening of the longitudinal arch and because the plantar surface of the foot is larger, gait economy is diminished. The patient tries to compensate for the longer anterior foot lever by adopting a more flat-footed gait, quite apart from the fact that the valgus foot in any case has a tendency to increased abduction.

The *rocker-bottomed foot* is the most severe form of contracted planovalgus foot and is characterised by a convex longitudinal arch along the sole of the foot. Typically, callouses form medially, toward the head of the talus; these are generally tender. Discounting the congenital valgus foot (which is not under discussion here and is also not a candidate for correction with orthopedic footwear), it is generally adults who develop a rocker-bottomed foot.

As has been outlined previously, basically the same principle of support under the sustentaculum tali obtains in contracted valgus foot. This relieves pressure on other parts of the foot and has the result of alleviating the symptom complex. Inserts are normally sufficient. However, if longitudinal arch flattening is considerable, and management would be more comfortable, orthopedic shoes are also indicated.

> Rx: One pair of made-to-measure corrective metal inserts with support for the sustentaculum tali and a recess for the plantar surface under the great toe.
> Diagnosis: Contracted planovalgus feet.

Where appropriate, and especially if the contractures and deformities are not quite so pronounced, inserts made of leather-lined cork may also be adequate to meet the need.

If there is some real prospect of the valgus deformity responding to correction, the recommended orthopedic footwear should be low shoes which afford support and relieve pressure.

> Rx: One pair of low orthopedic shoes (made to measure) to support the foot and relieve pressure. Medially displaced and flared buffer heel, stiffened shoe bottom and compensatory support under the sustentaculum tali incorporating a metatarsal bar.
> Diagnosis: Contracted planovalgus foot.

In the case of the completely convex rocker-bottomed foot, the principal task is to compensate for tenderness caused by the fallen longitudinal arch and for the unphysiological stress on parts of the plantar surface. The shoe waist must be absolutely stable and this can be achieved using a (cradle-shaped) wedge heel. Here, too, a low shoe is sufficient. The impaired mobility of the tarsal joints may be corrected using a metatarsal bar in cases where the wedge heel is not to be cradle-shaped.

Where the wedge heel and metatarsal bar merge with each other, the shoe bottom assumes an arched shape rather like the foot of a cradle. This prompted Henkel to name this design the cradle shoe (see Fig. 18). The centre of the arc of the sole should be located approximately at the midpoint of the thigh (see 3.3.4).

Rx: One pair of made-to-measure low orthopedic shoes to relieve pressure. With an elastic compensatory support, a full-length crepe sole and a wedge heel which is continuous with the metatarsal bar (Henkel's cradle shoe).

Diagnosis: Contracted rocker-bottomed foot.

5.1.7 Splayfoot

Generally, splayfoot is not encountered in isolation but in conjunction with another foot deformity, usually with pes planovalgus, or sometimes pes cavus. When accompanied by planotransversus foot, splayfoot stems in part from the fact that rollover occurs primarily along the medial border of the foot. This causes the first ray to bend in supination and, as a secondary result, the adjacent metatarsal heads assume a deeper position than normal.

Splayfoot occurring in conjunction with planotransversus foot requires all the management techniques described earlier (see 5.1.6.1), and a metatarsal pad may be prescribed in addition. Splayfoot in the context of pes equinoexcavatus is essentially part of the overall complex of the cavus foot and has been dealt with in the appropriate section (see 5.1.1).

Splayfoot in isolation is quite a rare phenomenon. However, splayfoot may be the single or principal cause of foot discomfort, and in such circumstances it requires preferential treatment.

A distinction is drawn between contracted splayfoot and another form which is still susceptible to passive correction.

5.1.7.1 Passively Correctable Splayfoot

Inserts and modifications to the retail shoe are more effective here than orthopedic shoes. The latter are generally only indicated where there is concurrent planovalgus/planotransversus foot, i.e. particularly when other orthopedic elements are also to be accommodated.

In cases where splayfoot flattening is simple to rectify, a corrective *splayfoot pad* should be incorporated in the retail shoe. As pointed out previously, the pad should be positioned immediately behind the metatarsal heads, and its height must be determined by the degree of flattening and discomfort.

Splayfoot corsets (still used fairly commonly) are not only uncomfortable, but may sometimes even be harmful if the bandage slips about on the foot and exerts bending forces at points where these may be painful.

If pain cannot be abolished despite correction, or perhaps because the deformity has already persisted for a fairly long period, then the *Marquardt horseshoe bar* is indicated. However, this can only be effective if the outsole is made of leather and the bottom filler is not too hard. Its particular function is to relieve pressure on the metatarsal heads during standing.

The remarks concerning inserts for planotransversus feet also apply here, but the metatarsal pad may be used in addition.

Rx: One pair of corrective planovalgus/planotransversus inserts made of metal (or leather-lined cork) with support under the sustentaculum tali and a metatarsal pad.
Diagnosis: Planovalgus/planotransversus feet.

5.1.7.2 Contracted Splayfoot

The main task here is to support and, where appropriate, provide soft padding for the painful metatarsal heads. In this case, too, the support function is performed by the *metatarsal pad: however, this should not be too high* because it is not in fact intended to have a corrective action. It must also be broad enough to distribute the ground reactive force over a sufficiently wide area.

If all the metatarsal heads are tender, a stepped insole is appropriate with the step positioned directly behind the joint line.

The splayfoot pad may also be accommodated as a modification to the retail shoe, but it is better to build it on to the insert.

In severe pain under the metatarsal heads, improvement can often be achieved by fitting a lateral outsole wedge.

Rx: One pair of metal (or leather-lined cork) supportive inserts, made to measure, with a fairly broad metatarsal pad of medium height.
Diagnosis: Planovalgus feet with contracted splayfeet.

Where the insert is to relieve pressure, the following prescription is recommended:

Rx: One pair of pressure-relieving leather-lined cork inserts, made to measure, with an insole with a transverse step behind the metatarsal heads. Good support for the sustentaculum tali.

Diagnosis: Painful planovalgus/planotransversus feet.

An orthopedic shoe is indicated when contracted splayfoot is accompanied by a planovalgus foot which could otherwise only be corrected with difficulty. The prescription should then be written as on page 63 ff.; the splayfoot pad is built on to the compensatory support.

Preference should also be given to an orthopedic shoe when the entire plantar surface of the foot is tender. In such circumstances, the recommendation is for a moulded insole of the type also used for feet deformed by chronic arthritis (see below).

5.1.8 The Deformed Foot
in Chronic Rheumatoid Arthritis

The foot in chronic rheumatoid arthritis is usually not only considerably deformed (splayfoot, hallux valgus, fibular deviations or clawing of the small toes, mutilating destruction of the metatarsophalangeal joints), but is also extremely tender and painful on movement as a result of inflammation and joint changes. It is this pain in particular which is generally so troublesome to the patient with rheumatoid arthritis and, in medical care terms, the deformities themselves may assume only secondary importance. Soft and extensive support for the entire plantar surface of the foot, using an insole moulded exactly to the contours of the patient's foot, is then the only means of alleviating this discomfort. However, although pain may be alleviated, greater force then has to be expended on walking and the gait becomes less elastic. A rocker bar will compensate for the reduced mobility of the metatarsophalangeal joints, but inevitably results in stiffening of the shoe bottom. Here again, the correct bottom filler is therefore vitally important, and the material selected needs to be especially elastic and soft. A wedge heel will relieve pressure on the tarsal joints. Henkel's cradle shoe may also be employed to advantage here. Very painful metatarsophalangeal joints should be supported with soft material; however, a harder material may be used for the midfoot and hindfoot.

Rx: One pair of low orthopedic shoes, made to measure (or plaster cast), with moulded insole incorporated into the compensatory support, concealed rocker bar, stiffened shoe bottom, wedge heel and bottom filler

made of soft and elastic material. Wedge heels designed as buffer heels.
Diagnosis: Deformed, tender foot in chronic rheumatoid arthritis.

Where the foot is not excessively tender, a stepped insole should be prescribed, with soft, pressure-relieving material for the metatarsophalangeal joints and harder material for the midfoot and hindfoot.

Rx: One pair of low orthopedic shoes, made to measure (or plaster cast), with stepped insole affording soft, pressure-relieving support for the metatarsophalangeal joints while the hindfoot rests on more solid material. Surface bar. Buffer heels.
Diagnosis: Deformed foot in chronic rheumatoid arthritis.

5.1.9 Claw Toes and Hammer Toes

The majority of such deformities can be adequately treated by modifying standard retail shoes. A *metatarsal pad* which stretches the aponeurosis commencing at the metatarsophalangeal joints will cause them to plantar flex. A *rocker bar* will facilitate rollover, and *felt ring pads* placed against the extensor aspects of the interphalangeal joints (and especially surrounding any callosities there) will exert cushioning and corrective effects simultaneously. A *roughened whole-length sock* will reduce the risk of foot slippage and prevent the toes from jarring painfully against the toe-end of the shoe.

Rx: Build a metatarsal pad into existing retail shoes. Insert a roughened whole-length sock and fit surface rocker bar (not too high).
Diagnosis: Claw toes.

Although orthopedic shoes may afford additional comfort, their prescription is in most instances a form of overtreatment. Where they are prescribed, however, the toe space should be enlarged and hammer toes (where present) should be supported with soft material.

Rx: One pair of made-to-measure orthopedic shoes with enlarged toe space, roughened whole-length sock with metatarsal pad, concealed rocker bar and soft cushioning for the tips of the toes.
Diagnosis: Painful and partially contracted claw toes.

5.1.10 Hallux Rigidus

The degenerative changes in the metatarsophalangeal joint of the great toe not only clearly impair the mobility of this joint, which is important for roll-over, but are also extremely painful. In functional mechanical terms, the anterior lever of the foot is lengthened because movements are now conducted mainly through the interphalangeal joint of the great toe. In addition, there is pressure discomfort caused by the shoe upper.

Consequently, corrective footwear must seek to *shorten this anterior lever* and, as far as possible, to eliminate pressure on the metatarsophalangeal joint caused by the shoe upper.

In principle, hallux rigidus can almost invariably be treated by modifying the retail shoe, where necessary also using metal inserts. The apex of the rocker bar in this case should lie beneath the sesamoid bones, but there should be no rocker material under the great toe itself.

Rx: Surface rocker bar with metal stiffening of the medial shoe bottom left.
Diagnosis: Hallux rigidus, left.

A cardinal feature of the insert should be a medial flange extending as far as the distal phalanx of the hallux. The orthopedic shoe can also alleviate the tenderness of the metatarsophalangeal joint if the upper is made of soft leather and if the toe space is enlarged.

Rx: One pair of made-to-measure low orthopedic shoes with a compensatory support which has a high rocker bar left and special support at the calcaneus. Buffer heel, enlarged toe space, soft upper leather and stiffened sole.
Diagnosis: Hallux rigidus, left.

5.1.11 Hallux Valgus

Hallux valgus is almost always accompanied by pes planovalgus or planotransversus, and these conditions should be treated accordingly. Reduction of the pressure caused by the shoe upper on the medial aspect of the metatarsophalangeal joint of the great toe can, in fact, only be achieved with an orthopedic shoe. Where hallux valgus is accompanied by pes planovalgus or planotransversus, it is essential that orthopedic shoes be constructed on the same principles as for pes planovalgus (see 5.1.6) or for splayfoot/planotransversus foot (see 5.1.7). Such shoes may be supportive or pressure-relieving or they may have a moulded insole, as in chronic rheumatoid arthritis (see 5.1.8). In each of these cases, enlargement of the upper over the medial joint line should also be prescribed.

5.2 Arthrodesis and Equinus

The prime task of the shoe in arthrodesis or ankylosis is to compensate as far as possible for the loss of mobility. This section will deal firstly with joint positions which are also achieved by surgery, and then with equinus foot.

5.2.1 Arthrodesis of Ankle Joint

In this case the ideal position is around the neutral position, i.e. when the lower leg is roughly at right angles to the foot. Recently, it has become favoured in male patients to position the foot in mild calcaneus (approximately 5°). Where there is leg inequality, the foot should be brought into mild equinus to create some degree of compensation.

The shoe which is designed to compensate for immobility in the ankle joint is generally the rocker-sole shoe. This is constructed as a low shoe and comprises the following four elements:

1. round-edge heel
2. metatarsal bar
3. wedge heel (preferably a heel with central waist support) and
4. non-slip sole

The height of rollover is adjusted to form an arc, the centre of which is located at the knee joint. The metatarsal bar should be moved back slightly so as to facilitate rollover and relieve pressure on the tarsal joints. However, the further back the metatarsal bar is moved, the less distance there is between it and the round-edge heel. In certain circumstances, therefore, it can be replaced by a cradle-shaped wedge heel. The metatarsal bar shortens the stand of the shoe and increases the risk of slipping. As a result the gait becomes more staccato. If the metatarsal bar is moved backwards, it is necessary to stiffen the shoe waist, ideally using a heel with a central waist support because this increases the non-slip properties of the shoe. The throat of the shoe should be extended towards the toe area to permit easy entry of the foot into the shoe.

Rx: One rocker-sole shoe (low shoe) with metatarsal bar moved back slightly, round-edge heel with central waist support, non-slip sole left and extended throat of shoe to permit easy entry.
Diagnosis: Ankylosis (following arthrodesis) of the left ankle joint.

5.2.2 Arthrodesis of Tarsal Joints

Generally, this causes only slight pain and minimal functional deficit. Consequently, simple modifications to the retail shoe are sufficient. A metatarsal bar moved backwards or a cradle-shaped wedge heel are in fact totally adequate and they also prevent painful bending of those joints which are still intact.

5.2.3 Arthrodesis of Metatarsophalangeal and Interphalangeal Joints

Ideally, the metatarsophalangeal joints should be stiffened in 20–25° dorsiflexion because this presents the least obstacle to rollover. The middle and distal phalanges should be stiffened in the extensor position.

In principle, the same measures apply here as already outlined for hallux rigidus (see 5.1.10). A surface rocker bar with metal stiffening of the medial sole is quite adequate in arthrodesis of the metatarsophalangeal joint of the hallux. If several metatarsophalangeal joints are stiffened, the entire shoe sole should be reinforced with a metal insert, and here too the surface rocker bar is effective in promoting rollover.

5.2.4 Arthrodesis of Knee Joint

The ideal position for stiffening is in 5–10° flexion. Generally, a shortening of up to 2 cm (0.8 inches) is felt to be beneficial for the swing phase. However, because the patient normally raises the pelvis on the same side when bringing the stiff leg forward, this rule may not necessarily apply. It merely implies that leg inequality of up to 2 cm (0.8 inches) does not require compensation. If the inequality is greater, a heel raise combined with a metatarsal bar will adequately compensate for inequality of up to 5 cm (2 inches).

5.2.5 Equinus

In contradistinction to foot-drop, the term equinus is used to designate impaired mobility in the ankle joint in which the foot can no longer be raised, even passively, above the neutral position (in which the foot is at right angles to the lower leg). In equinus, the longitudinal arch of the foot is generally more pronounced than normal, and there is usually also a valgus or varus deformity of the heel.

In terms of functional mechanics, severe equinus is characterised by the fact that the weight-bearing surface of the sole of the foot is reduced to the area under the metatarsal heads. Consequently, rollover is also only possible via the ball of the foot and the toes, and stride length is shortened, as with a raised shoe heel.

In the provision of footwear for this condition, the extent of equinus is not determined using the angle which the foot assumes in relation to the lower leg during maximum plantar flexion. Instead, with the patient standing erect and with simultaneous compensation provided for the other limb, a block is used to measure the distance between the calcaneus and the ground when the pelvis is levelled.

5.2.5.1 General Principles of Management

1. The prime objective must be to distribute load-bearing as far as possible over the entire sole of the foot: to this end, the calcaneus should be padded firmly and relatively deeply on the compensatory support.

2. Any relative limb shortness of the other leg should be corrected.

3. When measuring differences in leg length using the block technique, the principles of sagittal (lateral) perpendicular construction must be remembered. In equinus, therefore, the perpendicular from the hip joint should generally pass just in front of the knee joint axis during standing and continue behind the metatarsal heads.

4. Any residual potential for active plantar flexion should be exploited provided that this is not painful. Consequently, the most flexible shoe possible

should be prescribed. The heel selected should be the lowest one permitting exploitation of full plantar flexion, i. e. equinus is then measured with the foot in maximum dorsiflexion.

5. A toe grip bar with horizontal support padding for the toes is more important than a metatarsal pad which usually only causes unnecessary discomfort and should therefore be dispensed with.

6. Where there is extensor impairment of the knee joint, the equinus foot must not be fully compensated because this would exert a flexor effect on the knee joint during the load-bearing phase and there would be no locking action.

7. Severe equinus foot can be managed more effectively with an internal shoe and extremely severe equinus (greater than 7 cm or 2.8 inches) should be treated like major leg inequality.

8. Conversely, where the condition is less pronounced (up to approximately 2.5 cm or 1 inch), modifications to the retail shoe are sufficient.

9. Where the equinus foot is to be corrected in the shoe, compensation under the calcaneus should not be complete so that the patient's bodyweight will press the calcaneus downwards.

10. In fact, the calcaneus should only be raised if the leg in question is also short. Otherwise, compensation of the sound limb would become too clumsy. And this is really the full extent to which the equinus foot can be managed with orthopedic footwear. Surgical intervention is the appropriate treatment for the more severe forms of equinus without leg shortening. In such cases, the provision of orthopedic footwear would be a form of overtreatment because the sound limb would also require compensation in a way which would be medically unacceptable because of the resultant positional anomaly. And then there are cosmetic considerations. Nevertheless, such measures are sometimes needed, either because surgery is flatly refused or is untenable on general medical grounds. For this reason, and because they provide characteristic illustrations of the general principles pertaining to the management of the equinus foot, these measures will be described more fully here. Where leg inequality is additionally present, those principles should be applied which relate to the correction of leg inequality in isolation.

In the context of orthopedic footwear provision, it is beneficial to differentiate between the mild (up to 2.5 cm/1 inch), moderate (up to 5 cm/2 inches), severe (up to 7 cm/2.8 inches) and extremely severe (greater than 7 cm/2.8 inches) forms of equinus foot. These distinctions apply when the ankle joint is completely stiff. Where some mobility remains, length deficit is measured with the foot in maximum dorsiflexion.

5.2.5.2 Mild Equinus Foot without Leg Inequality with Arthrodesis of Ankle Joint

Modifications to both retail shoes are generally sufficient in such cases. The situation is the same as for the moderate equinus foot, only less severe.

The following prescription may be recommended in equinus of 2.5 cm (1 inch):

Rx: Raise left heel 3 cm (1.2 inches), compensatory material 0.5 cm (0.2 inches) thick under left calcaneus, surface metatarsal bar 1 cm (0.4 inches) high. Full-length midsole (0.5 cm/0.2 inches thick) right. Raise right heel 1 cm (0.4 inches), compensatory material 0.5 cm (0.2 inches) thick under right calcaneus. Surface rocker bar 0.5 cm (0.2 inches) high, right.

Diagnosis: Mild equinus foot, left.

5.2.5.3 Moderate Equinus Foot without Leg Inequality with (Complete) Arthrodesis of Ankle Joint

Clinical situation:

1. Affected leg is relatively longer.
2. Anterior lever arm (i.e. effective mechanical foot length) is markedly shortened.
3. During rollover, load-bearing is displaced forward towards the tip of the foot.
4. No residual movement in the ankle joint.

Shoe management principles:

1. Correct the shortness of the sound limb.
2. Make up foot length by means of a foot prosthesis with either:
   a) a stiffened sole which extends from the joint line to the calcaneus as for the healthy foot or
   b) a stiffened tongue which extends as far as the anterior edge of the foot prosthesis.
3. Fit an orthopedic bar (not too far back, if prescribed at all).
4. A metatarsal bar will act as a substitute for ankle joint mobility, but then the entire shoe bottom should be stiffened to prevent the shoe from bending upwards.
5. Pad and support the calcaneus deeply and firmly to reduce the risk of slippage.
6. Where necessary, fit a buffer heel to shorten slightly the relatively longer posterior lever arm and to increase rollover at the heel.

7. Where necessary, fit a toe grip bar or Eisenmann strap to prevent dead
   movement of the foot inside the shoe.

Rx: One pair of orthopedic laced ankle boots (plaster cast), with support
to compensate for inequality of ... cm (or: compensatory support which
raises the calcaneus by ... cm), with toe grip bar, sole stiffened as far as the
joint line and Eisenmann strap (or: with total sole stiffening, metatarsal bar
and stiffened anterior tongue). Raise plus rocker bar to compensate for
short right leg.
Diagnosis: Arthrodesis of the left ankle joint in equinus.

5.2.5.4 Severe Equinus Foot without Leg Inequality with Arthrodesis of Ankle Joint

The clinical situation and the principles of orthopedic shoe management
are essentially the same as for moderate equinus, only more comprehensive
(in certain respects). The provision of an internal shoe would therefore appear
appropriate.

Rx: One internal shoe, prepared in hard foam casting resin from a plaster
cast, for the left leg to give ... cm compensation, and shock-absorbent material under the calcaneus. Compensation for short right leg.
Diagnosis: Severe equinus foot left with arthrodesis of the ankle joint.

5.2.5.5 Extremely Severe Equinus Foot

In theory, this condition should be catered for in accordance with the principles used to correct leg inequality greater than 12 cm (4.8 inches), i.e. with a
type of lower leg prosthesis. However, this would merely further increase the
leg lengthening due to equinus. In such circumstances, therefore, a Körting
shoe prosthesis might possibly be more appropriate (Fig. 45). This incorporates
a stiff upright leather sheath, the bed of which surrounds and supports the tar-
sals, and a foot prosthesis over which a retail shoe may even be worn.

However, such forms of management for the severe and extremely severe
equinus foot border on the ridiculous and are in fact totally unrealistic. Quite
apart from cosmetic considerations, the compensation necessary for the sound
leg would have a harmful anatomical effect, resulting in excessive limb lengthening and gait unsteadiness on both sides. Wherever possible, corrective surgery is absolutely essential to remedy the situation.

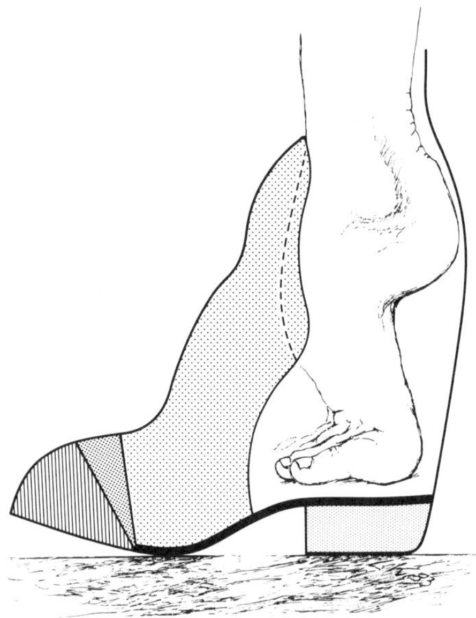

Fig. 45. Körting shoe prosthesis

5.2.5.6 Spastic Equinus Foot

The guidelines given for the non-spastic equinus foot also apply in principle to the spastic equinus foot in cases where surgery has been refused. However, where passive dorsiflexion produces a marked pathological increase in muscle tone, footwear should never attempt to correct the equinus foot, but simply to compensate for the deformity. In spasticity due to infantile cerebral palsy, the affected leg is generally as much as 2 cm (0.8 inches) shorter than the healthy leg. In such circumstances the equinus position should also be exploited to the full to compensate for the leg inequality and the calcaneus should be supported accordingly. It is also beneficial to retain (or even to create) an overall 1 cm to 1.5 cm (0.4 to 0.6 inch) inequality to allow the affected leg to swing through more efficiently.

The flaccid equinus foot (foot-drop) is dealt with in the section on peroneal nerve paralysis (see 5.5.1).

5.3 Immobilisation of Painful Joints

Generally, it is the final phases of the range of movement which are particularly sensitive in a joint which is painful to move. Such joints should therefore ideally be immobilised in an intermediate position so that any residual movement inside the shoe which cannot be totally eliminated occurs in the less sensitive range. This position should be established in each case by the physician and the information passed on to the shoemaker.

5.3.1 Immobilisation of Ankle Joint

Rabl's rigid rocker-sole shoe (Fig. 46) is ideal for this purpose. In this shoe a round-ankle stiffener (stiffened tongue in front combined with a high ankle stiffener behind) serves to immobilise the ankle joint. A peroneal iron lends further reinforcement to the high ankle stiffener, and a round-edge heel and metatarsal bar together ensure correct rollover. The metatarsal bar is usually

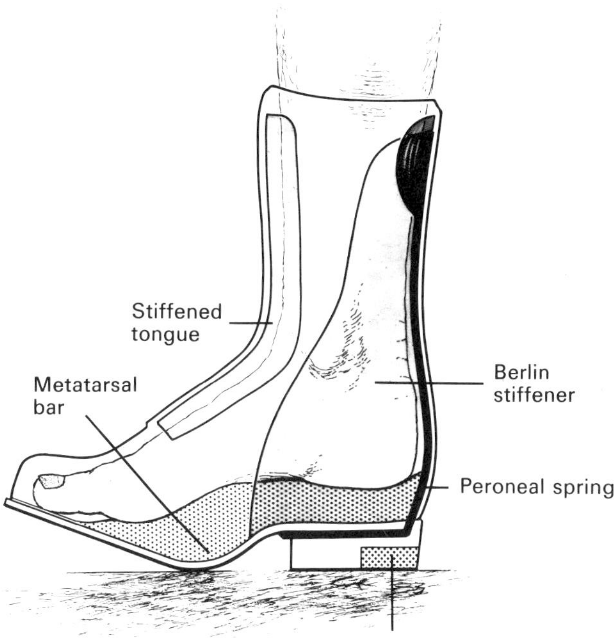

Fig. 46. Rabl rigid rocker-sole shoe

built into the compensatory support (internal bar) and forms an arc, the centre of which is located approximately at the knee joint. Since the contact surface between ground and shoe is reduced in relative terms, a heel with a central waist support is recommended to improve the non-slip characteristics of the shoe. The shoe on the healthy side is raised so that the leg becomes 0.5 cm (0.2 inches) longer. Even when constructed by a shoemaker who has a special regard for cosmetic considerations, the rigid rocker-sole shoe invariably appears clumsy and never makes the act of walking unobtrusive.

Rx: One Rabl rigid rocker-sole shoe left (with round-ankle stiffener, Heidelberg angle, round-edge heel with central waist support and metatarsal bar built into the compensatory support), compensation to make the right leg 0.5 cm (0.2 inches) longer than the left.
Diagnosis: Left ankle joint painful on movement.

5.3.2 Immobilisation of Tarsal Joints

The measures described on page 64 f. also apply here and will not be repeated. However, if discomfort is not alleviated as a result, the rigid rocker-sole shoe will generally afford greater relief.

The principles outlined on page 63 f. clearly demonstrate why the following prescription is recommended when a poorly healed calcaneal fracture remains painful on movement:

Rx: One pair of orthopedic shoes, made to measure, with 4.5 cm (1.8 inch) high buffer heels on both shoes, flared medially and laterally, with stiffened shoe bottom left, concealed metatarsal bar moved back slightly, round-heel counter to give mediolateral stability, a soft upper which fits the metatarsus snugly, and compensatory support with padding under the sustentaculum tali.
Diagnosis: Poorly healed calcaneal fracture left.

A cradle-shaped wedge heel may be recommended here in particular instead of the metatarsal bar.

This prescription could also be used in tarsal arthrosis. In calcaneal fractures, laced ankle boots are sometimes more effective because their heel counters extend over a larger area and the foot is generally gripped more firmly.

Rabl's rigid rocker-sole shoe, which also immobilises the ankle joint, generally becomes superfluous with the above measures which can be varied to meet the requirements of each individual case.

5.3.3 Immobilisation of Metatarsophalangeal Joints

The remarks concerning hallux rigidus also apply here (see 5.1.10). If the desired objective remains unachieved, the further advantages possibly to be conferred by a moulded insole should be considered (see 3.1.3), particularly in cases where all the metatarsophalangeal joints are painful.

However, a stepped insole may also be beneficial in individual cases, because less energy is expended during walking than with a shoe containing a moulded insole.

5.4 Leg Inequality and Leg Deformities

5.4.1 Compensation for the Short Leg

The short leg is probably less amenable to a standard set of orthopedic footwear rules than any other anomaly. There are several reasons for this. Inequality of leg length varies from patient to patient and, for that reason alone, necessitates fundamentally different management principles. In addition, anatomical features of the joints or of sections of the extremities may display marked differences. And finally, cosmetic and functional requirements are occasionally at odds and yet have to be reconciled by compromise. No catalogue of rules could possibly take account of all wishes, potential combinations and anatomical details.

Nevertheless, certain "universal" features and *management principles* may be listed here:

1. Any relatively pronounced shortening should be accommodated by positioning the foot in equinus. In functional mechanical terms, the anterior lever of the foot becomes shorter as the degree of equinus increases, and this in turn has the following results:
   a) The more the foot is brought into equinus, the higher the calcaneus is raised (by about 1.5 cm to 2 cm/0.6 to 0.8 inches in extreme circumstances) (Fig. 47). The compensatory support under the calcaneus therefore needs to be raised by the same amount. Furthermore, when determining the amount of raise required to compensate for the inequality,

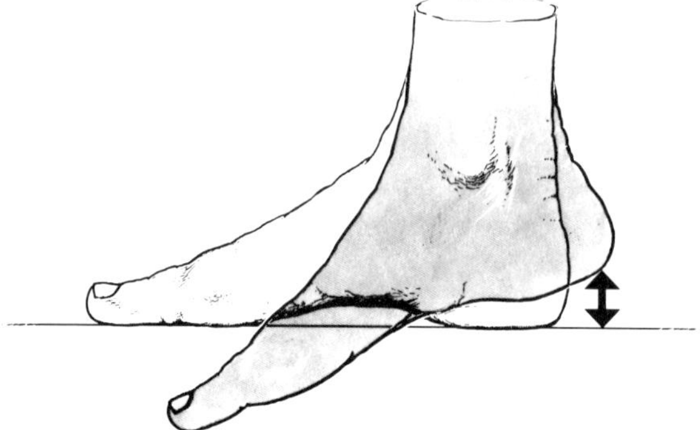

Fig. 47. Raising the calcaneus by bringing the foot into equinus

separate measurements should be taken under the calcaneus and the metatarsal heads.
  b) The markedly shortened anterior lever should be supplemented with a foot prosthesis so that the front part of the shoe appears balanced. In major leg inequality, this prosthesis-like filler should have a spring-loaded joint which stretches the front part of the shoe bottom after toe-off (Fig. 48). This joint, which is at right angles to the direction of travel, should be

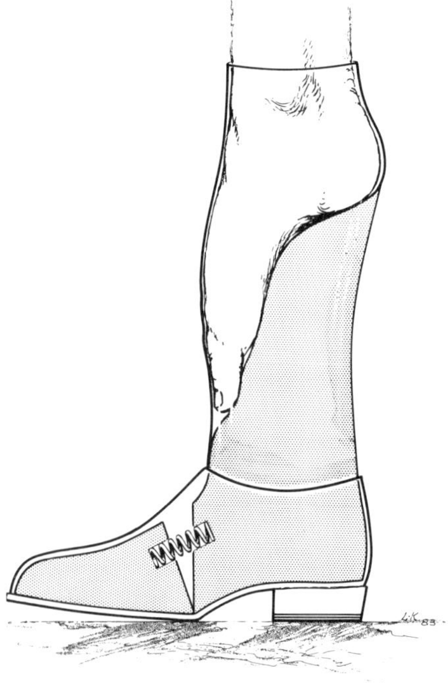

Fig. 48. Prosthetic foot filler with spring-loaded joint (from Marquardt)

positioned precisely at the anterior limit of the shoe waist and slightly behind the joint line.

c) The shoe bottom should always be stiffened. When using a jointed foot
prosthesis, the stiffening should extend forward from the back of the shoe
as far as the anterior limit of the waist, i.e. to behind the joint line.

2. The foot should not slide off its support easily. This may be achieved in
the following ways:

a) The calcaneus should be deeply padded, but not excessively so because
this will merely cause discomfort.

b) A toe grip bar is usually appropriate, but not a metatarsal pad because
this would cause pain.

c) In addition, the dorsum of the metatarsus should always be gripped
firmly by the upper.

3. The foot should only be brought into equinus to the point at which the
knee remains slightly flexed during standing. This can be achieved by ensuring
that the lateral perpendicular passes from the hip joint, slightly behind the
knee joint, in front of the lateral malleolar tip and thus to the ground.

4. Where ankle joint mobility is to be preserved, the calcaneus should not be
raised by more than 4 cm (1.6 inches) relative to the plantar surface of the joint
line. In other words, once the calcaneus has been raised by 4 cm (1.6 inches),
the plantar surface at the joint line and that under the calcaneus should then be
raised further by equal amounts, provided that further compensation is not dispensed with altogether. For example, in leg shortening of 6 cm (2.4 inches),
support would have to be 6 cm (2.4 inches) high under the calcaneus compared
with 2 cm (0.8 inches) under the ball of the foot. The toes should not be supported in excessive dorsiflexion if they are to play an active part in rollover.

5. All dead movement inside the shoe must be eliminated and the measures
listed under 2 above will largely achieve this. A stiffened tongue would reinforce this effect, but is only indicated if there is to be no further movement in
the ankle joint: this is one of its disadvantages. A second disadvantage of the
stiffened tongue is that it generally also requires a metatarsal bar, which in turn
presupposes a totally stiffened shoe bottom and renders impossible any joint-
like device in the toe filler. The following additional guidelines may also be
given.:

6. The greater the compensation required, the more the shoe bottom and heel
should be flared laterally (approximately 1 mm for every 1 cm of compensation). This recommendation has its basis in the fact that, during rollover, lateral

forces develop which could bend the shoe over. The lateral flare counteracts this tendency.

7. If there is already a prolonged history of pronounced shortening, initial management should not attempt to position the foot in full equinus or to provide full compensation, because both measures would cause discomfort, the former in the foot and the latter in the back.

8. Where cosmetic considerations demand particular attention, every centimeter should be compensated and the foot should be brought into full equinus and held in position with a bandage-like upper (MARQUARDT, 1965).

Marquardt also lists the following rules:

9. In the event of extensor and flexor contracture in the hip joint, shortening should be compensated until the patient is able to stand comfortably and lock both knees fully.

10. Discrepancies in leg length in a patient with genu valgum should not be fully compensated; a discrepancy of 1 to 1.5 cm (0.4 to 0.6 inches) should be left uncompensated.

11. The same applies in stiffening of the knee joint.

12. Finally, the following general rules may be given:
a) Inequalities up to 3 to 4 cm (1.2 to 1.6 inches) can be treated by modifying the retail shoe.
b) Inequalities up to about 8 cm (3.2 inches) require an orthopedic shoe.
c) Inequalities up to about 12 cm (4.8 inches) require an internal shoe.
d) Inequalities in excess of 12 cm (4.8 inches) require a shoe prosthesis or an O'Connor boot.

All the measurements given here refer to inequalities in adults but, scaled down appropriately, they also apply in children. It is axiomatic in children, however, that any inequality greater than 1 cm (0.4 inches) requires compensation, whereas in adults there is probably rather more room for discretion in individual cases.

5.4.1.1 Leg Inequality up to 3 to 4 cm (1.2 to 1.6 inches)

Depending on the degree of inequality, compensation may be effected with shoe modifications comprising the following elements (Fig. 49):

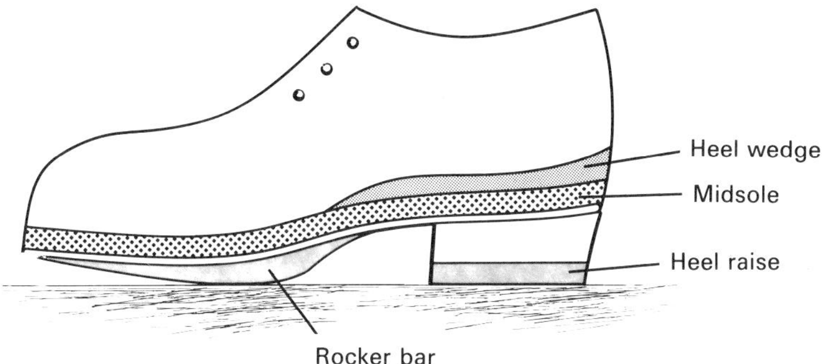

Fig. 49. Modifications to retail shoe in leg inequality up to 3–4 cm (1.2–1.6 inches)

1. Heel wedge (never higher than 1 cm/0.4 inches).
2. Midsole (approx. 0.5 cm/0.2 inches) between outsole and insole.
3. Heel raise up to 1 cm (0.4 inches).
4. Rocker bar of same height as shoe heel.
5. Flattening of contralateral heel (not more than 0.5 cm/0.2 inches).

All together, these elements give a maximum compensation of 3 cm (1.2 inches). Since a 2 cm (0.8 inch) difference in leg length can be ignored, a 5 cm (2 inch) inequality could theoretically be compensated in this way. However, the anatomical situation in each individual patient must always determine whether it is really legitimate to go as far as 5 cm (2 inches).

Care should therefore be taken to ensure that the shoe heel on the relatively longer side is not reduced excessively because the toe spring would become too large. Conversely, *a heel raise without an equally high rocker bar will reduce the toe spring.*

Rx: Compensate for shortening on left by modifying the retail shoe as follows: Add a 1 cm (0.4 inch) heel raise, surface rocker bar 1 cm (0.4 inches) high and a 0.5 cm (0.2 inch) midsole raise and glue in a 1 cm (0.4 inch) heel wedge. Reduce height of right heel by 0.5 cm (0.2 inches).
Diagnosis: Leg inequality (left) of 3 cm (1.2 inches).

It may also be necessary to fit a heel tab (by raising the top line at the back of the shoe) to prevent the calcaneus from slipping out of the shoe.

5.4.1.2 Leg Inequality up to 8 cm (3.2 inches)

An orthopedic laced ankle boot is indicated here for men: the boot should be made to measure or, if there is simultaneous foot deformity, prepared from a plaster cast. It should be remembered that the "sound shoe" also has a heel and an orthopedic bar. Compensation is thus only achieved by the height of the calcaneal support, irrespective of how much the foot is brought into equinus. The shoe should be fitted with the following orthopedic elements:

1. The height of the compensatory support under the calcaneus should be the same as the discrepancy in leg length. The calcaneus should be cupped relatively deeply to prevent the foot from slipping off the support. This can be achieved most effectively with:

2. A round-ankle stiffener which immobilises the ankle joint. Of course, this is not indicated where ankle joint movement is still required. In such cases,

3. The ball of the foot should also be raised on the compensatory support up to a height of 3 cm (1.2 inches) (i.e. in leg inequality of 7 cm/2.8 inches, then 7 cm/2.8 inches minus 4 cm/1.6 inches = 3 cm/1.2 inches). This also gives the shoe a somewhat clumsy appearance.

4. Where a round-ankle stiffener is used, the metatarsal bar should be about 1.5 cm (0.6 inches) high. This amount should not be subtracted from the height of the compensatory support under the calcaneus, but must be taken into account in the shoe heel.

5. The shoe should contain a flexible toe filler and

6. Either a stiffened sole which extends from the back of the shoe to the theoretical joint line of the healthy foot and causes the toe prosthesis to move via its leading edge, or a stiffened full-length sole where a round-ankle stiffener is prescribed.

7. A toe grip bar.

8. A buffer heel is also recommended and

9. Internal fastening (two broad pieces of leather, attached one at each side between the upper and the insole at the back of the shoe and exerting a firm grip on the metatarsus. These are then laced together at the front under the upper.)

10. A paralysis counter is indicated in cases where a round-ankle stiffener appears excessive, but where plantar movement in the ankle joint is not desired (Fig. 50).

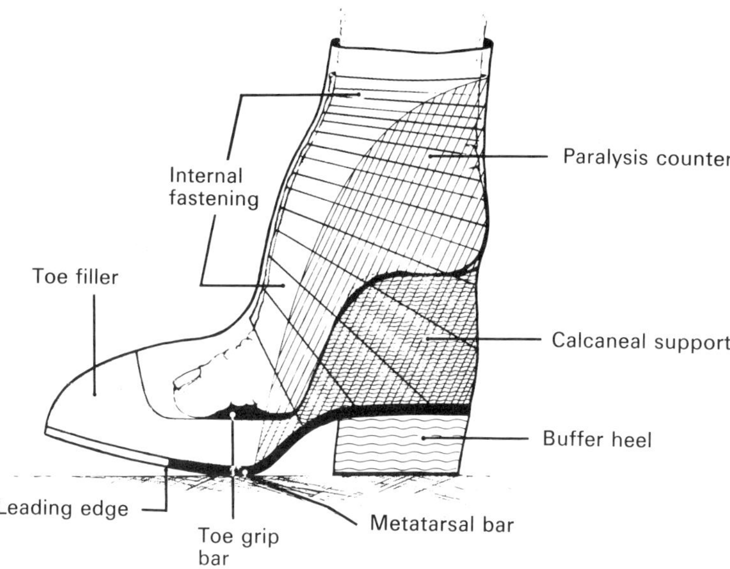

Fig. 50. Orthopedic shoe to accommodate leg inequality up to 8 cm (3.2 inches). (From Regenspurger)

Without a paralysis counter, the shoe upper should rise as far as the malleolus of the affected foot, provided that ankle joint movement is permitted.

Rx: One pair of orthopedic shoes, plaster cast, with internal fastening left, buffer heel, sole stiffened from rear forwards to in front of the metatarsal bar left and compensatory support left which raises the calcaneus by 7 cm (2.8 inches) and the ball of the foot by 3 cm (1.2 inches), and which incorporates a toe grip bar and a 1.5 cm (0.6 inch) metatarsal bar.
Diagnosis: Leg inequality (left) of 7 cm (2.8 inches).

In this case, therefore, movement in the ankle joint is still possible and desirable. For cosmetic reasons, female patients require an internal shoe of the type described for the compensation of leg inequality up to 12 cm (4.8 inches).

5.4.1.3 Leg Inequality up to 12 cm (4.8 inches)

In such cases it is generally no longer sufficient simply to bring the foot into equinus. Consequently, the ball of the foot invariably also needs to be raised, but only to a maximum height of 5 cm (2 inches). An internal shoe is indicated here and is ordered with an orthopedic made-to-measure shoe containing a toe filler. The ankle joint should be immobilised using a round-ankle stiffener and the compensatory material under the calcaneus may be as high as 12 cm (4.8 inches). The orthopedic shoe containing the internal shoe is constructed in essentially the same way as for leg inequality up to 7 cm (2.8 inches) but, in addition to the buffer heel, should also have shock-absorbent material under the cupped calcaneal support. The foot itself is fastened in an internal shoe made of casting resin or hard foam material (Fig. 51).

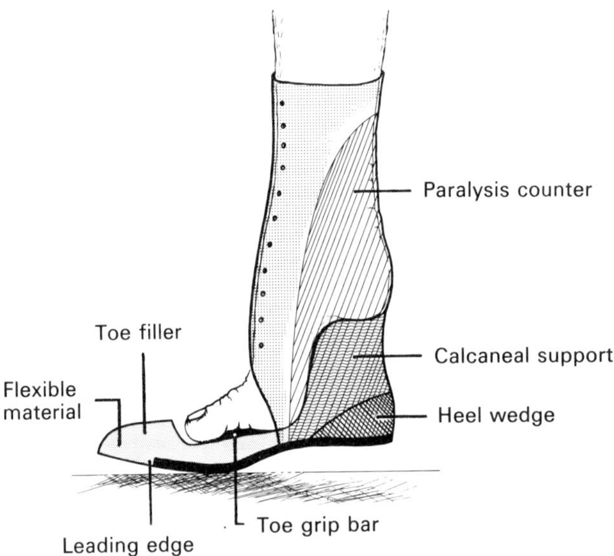

Fig. 51. Internal shoe to accommodate leg inequality up to 12 cm (4.8 inches). (From Regenspurger)

Rx: One internal shoe left made of hard foam/casting resin to give a 12 cm (4.8 inch) calcaneal raise with the foot in equinus. The internal shoe should have an upper height of 18 cm (7.2 inches) and should encase the forefoot as far as the metatarsophalangeal joints. Also, one orthopedic shoe left, including compensatory support with a 12 cm (4.8 inch) calcaneal raise, shock-absorbent heel wedge and toe grip bar; also with a toe filler, a round-ankle stiffener, a stiffened full-length sole with 5 cm (2 inch) raise for the ball of the foot and a 1.5 cm (0.6 inch) metatarsal bar. Made-to-measure shoe right with rocker bar.

Diagnosis: Leg inequality (left) of 12 cm (4.8 inches).

5.4.1.4 Leg Inequality in excess of 12 cm (4.8 inches)

Large inequalities of this kind can be accommodated in one of two ways:

1. By creating a support as for a prosthesis for a pointed lower-leg amputation stump.
2. By using an O'Connor boot.

The former alternative is really the province of the orthopedic technician and should be executed in accordance with the rules of lower-leg prosthesis construction. However, it should be mentioned that a shoe prosthesis of the Körting type (see Fig. 45), for example, is not so beneficial. Because the foot is in extreme equinus, bodyweight is transmitted to the metatarsal bones, causing the shearing forces to act on a relatively small area. This is not always tolerated without discomfort.

O'Connor Boot

The principle of the O'Connor boot has already been described on page 41. The more the foot is positioned at right angles to the lower leg, the more secure the entire shoe during walking. For cosmetic reasons, however, varying degrees of equinus have to be permitted sometimes as a compromise measure (Fig. 52). Because the design is virtually standard, the O'Connor boot is very simple to prescribe and is virtually synonymous with the specific diagnosis.

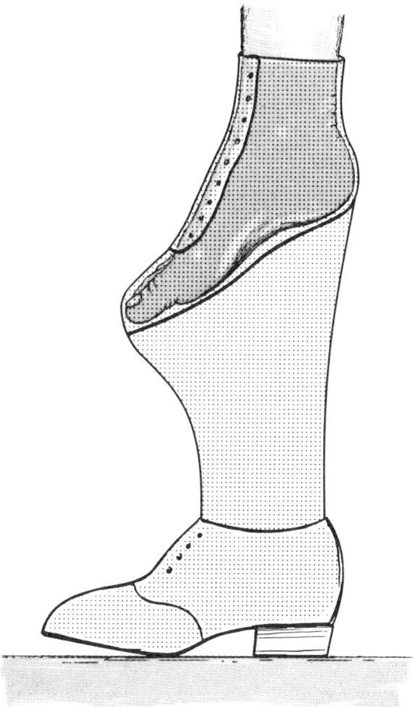

Fig. 52. O'Connor boot

Rx: One O'Connor boot left to compensate for a leg inequality of ... cm. Support foot in ...° equinus.
Diagnosis: Leg inequality (left) of ... cm.

5.4.2 Genu Valgum

Genu valgum in childhood is commonly associated with planotransversus feet. Since the weight line deviates from the perpendicular in this condition, the resultant pathological tangential and shearing forces further aggravate genu valgum and planotransversus feet (see Fig. 35).

Absolute adherence to the principles of perpendicular shoe construction is therefore essential and the sole of the shoe must be balanced to the weight-bearing surface of the foot. The heel should be supinated and the planotransversus foot should be treated as for the passively correctable form of that deformity (see 5.1.6.1). Almost invariably, this can be done simply by modifying the retail shoe. In children, a supination wedge should be incorporated into the shoe and the heel should have a medial flare. While genu valgum cannot be corrected in this way, it is nevertheless possible to minimise the forces which would further aggravate the deformity, thereby alleviating the discomfort caused. Where this is particularly pronounced, a medium-hard buffer heel is required.

5.4.3 Genu Varum

Genu varum in childhood is also generally associated with planotransversus feet. However, as already stated on page 50 in connection with the principles of perpendicular shoe construction, correction of the stance anomaly is now only partially possible because lateral flaring of the shoe sole and heel would exacerbate the foot deformity and cause greater discomfort. If these disadvantages prove acceptable, then the forces which continue to act on genu varum can be reduced somewhat by a lateral flare on a buffer heel.

There must remain some doubt concerning the benefits to be gained from lateral wedging of the shoe bottom and heel because this measure is hardly ever successful in correcting genu varum. Moreover, the resultant oblique angle of the ankle joint will expose it increasingly to unilateral forces which can only be deleterious in the long term.

In summary, any corrective footwear should be employed circumspectly in genu varum, and the benefits and disadvantages should be weighed with special care in each individual patient.

5.4.4 Genu Recurvatum

The management of genu recurvatum with corrective footwear alone is somewhat problematic. In most cases, genu recurvatum arises as a passive locking mechanism to replace extensor muscle action at the knee and to prevent flexion; as a result, the ligament apparatus becomes increasingly hyperextended. Orthopedic footwear is never adequate in severe cases of paralysis. However, in advanced hyperextension of the ligament apparatus, raising the heel may always be recommended to inhibit the locking effect on the knee joint. The heel raise should be adapted to suit the needs of the individual patient. Account must also be taken of the patient's comfort and some trial and error may therefore be necessary.

5.4.5 Elephantiasis

This pathological condition almost invariably requires orthopedic footwear because the unwieldy girth of the foot and lower leg prevents the patient from wearing retail shoes. Orthopedic footwear should then be constructed as ankle boots or half boots to give a snug fit at the foot and lower leg, to prevent the feet from slipping out and to eliminate leg constriction due to an excessively tight top line. Additional orthopedic elements may be incorporated in line with individual needs. Where pes planotransversus is present, for example, pressure-relieving or supportive measures should also be used to treat this condition in its own right. The upper should not be stiffened.

Rx: One pair of orthopedic half boots with front lacing and soft upper leather, made to measure.
Diagnosis: Bilateral elephantiasis.

Where appropriate, a side zip fastener may be fitted for cosmetic reasons.

5.5 Flaccid Paralysis

5.5.1 Peroneal Nerve Paralysis

This is one of the commonest of all types of paralysis. In motor neurone terms, the deep peroneal nerve supplies the extensor group of the lower leg. When this nerve is paralysed, dorsiflexion of the entire foot at the ankle joint and of the toes is no longer possible. Paralysis of the superficial peroneal nerve affects the peroneal group, which means that the foot can no longer be pronated.

Peroneal nerve paralysis is an impediment to walking primarily because the patient often stumbles over the dropped foot as the toes drag on the ground during ambulation.

This type of paralysis can be treated in three ways. Firstly, the foot may be dorsiflexed using strips of elastic. Secondly, dorsiflexion can be achieved using a metal or plastic spring which extends from the posterior aspect of the calf under the back of the heel and along the sole and which, because of its elasticity, raises the foot from underneath. Thirdly, a spiral spring may be fitted to a retail shoe.

The four approaches to the correction of peroneal nerve paralysis described below operate by one of these three principles.

1. A *spiral spring* may be fitted laterally as a modification to a retail ankle boot (high shoe); the spring acts to dorsiflex the front part of the foot (in front of the shoe heel). The disadvantage of this method is that the spiral spring is unsightly and may lose some elasticity with time. On the positive side, a spiral

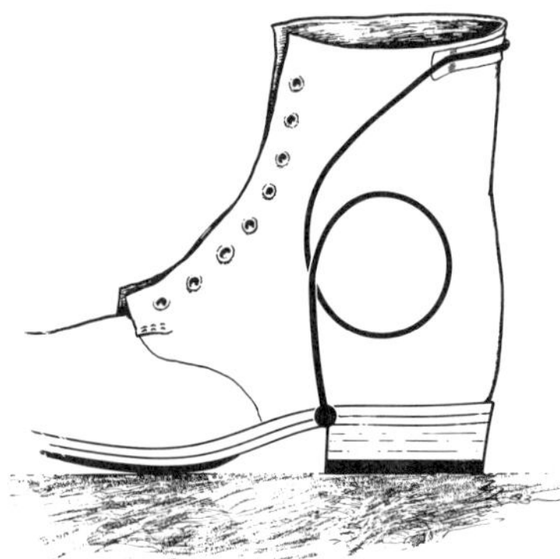

Fig. 53. Spiral spring fitted to retail shoe in peroneal nerve paralysis

spring is not only simple, but also extremely effective, restoring virtually normal gait in mild and moderate peroneal nerve paralysis (Fig. 53).

2. *Internal shoes* may utilise either elastic strips or a posterior angled stiffener. The *Breidbach bandage* functions on the first of these principles. It contains no stiffening element and can be worn easily under the patient's sock or stocking. Because it develops only minimal force, it is indicated exclusively in mild forms of peroneal nerve paralysis. However, it is particularly acceptable in cosmetic terms because it is virtually invisible. The Breidbach bandage incorporates a firm foot support which is attached to a type of peroneal spring and extends upwards behind the heel. The peroneal spring is also attached to elasticated strips which raise the foot additionally (Fig. 54).

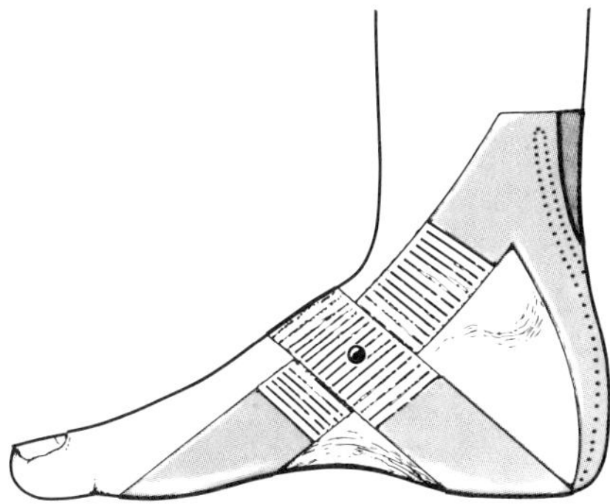

Fig. 54. Breidbach bandage for mild peroneal nerve paralysis

The *Kraus paralysis internal shoe* (Fig. 55) is constructed with a leather upper fastened with front lacing. The internal shoe contains an angled stiffening element which extends from the sole of the foot behind the heel and beyond the malleoli. This metal stiffening element bifurcates medially and laterally in the calcaneal region so as not to exert pressure on the Achilles tendon. The upper and stiffening element extend forward as far as the metatarsophalangeal joints.

This internal shoe is suitable for moderate paralysis and is also cosmetically acceptable. It generally also requires a made-to-measure shoe.

Of course, peroneal internal shoes also exist which operate on the same principle but extend higher (i.e. with an upper height of 18 cm/7.2 inches). This type of internal shoe also requires made-to-measure shoes.

3. *Toe-raising springs* also exert their action from behind and underneath the foot. They are casting resin angles comprising a profiled footplate and a spring which encases the posterior aspect of the calf (Fig. 56). The upper extremity of the toe-raising spring is attached to the lower leg by a calf band. However,

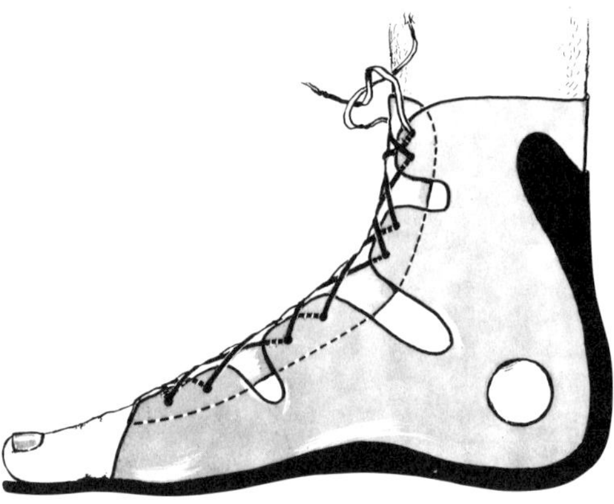

Fig. 55. Kraus internal shoe for moderate peroneal nerve paralysis

these toe-raising springs may also grip the foot like a stirrup (cf. the Lehneis spiral, Fig. 57) and spiral up round the lower leg. Additional advantages of the Lehneis spiral are that it exerts a pronating force (especially beneficial in paralysis also involving the deep peroneal nerve) and does not cause pressure on those points at the head of the fibula which are particularly sensitive for the peroneal nerve. The spiral is no more obtrusive than an angled toe-raising spring. When it is not load-bearing, the foot in a toe-raising spring may be in 5° plantar flexion (but no more). Care should be taken to check this in each instance.

A reasonably good gait pattern and, in particular, good rollover cannot always be achieved with a toe-raising spring alone. In such cases, a surface metatarsal bar fitted to a retail shoe, a slight heel raise (1–2 cm/0.4–0.8 inches) and a buffer heel are effective.

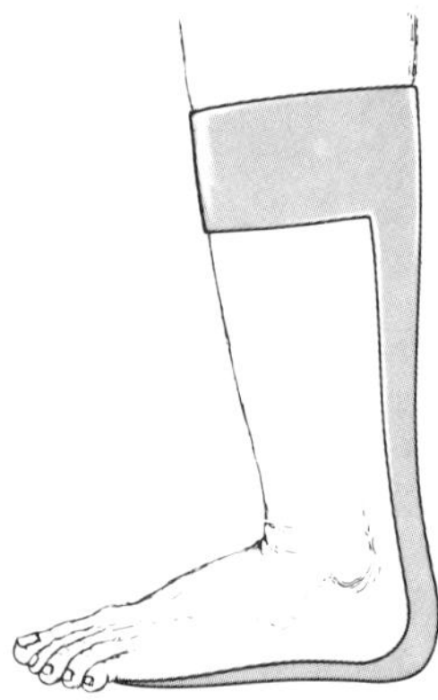

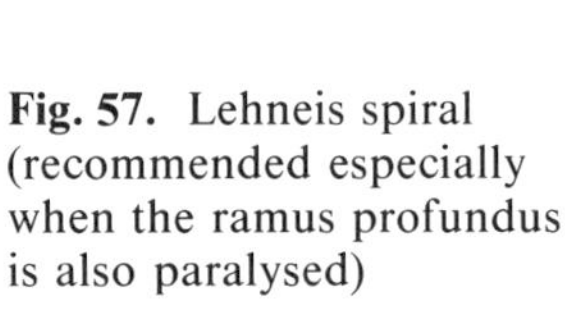

Fig. 56. Simple toe-raising spring for peroneal nerve paralysis

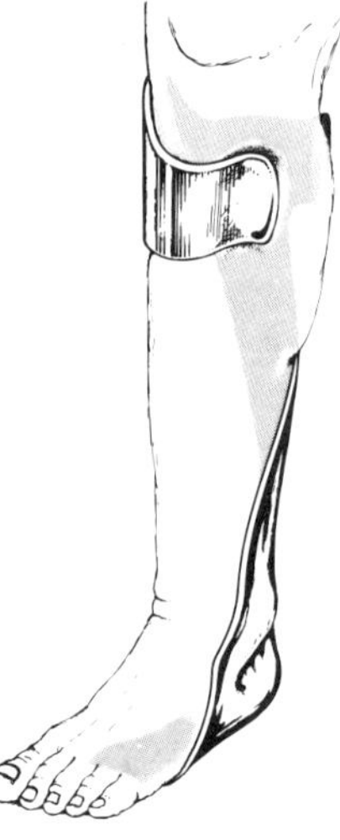

Fig. 57. Lehneis spiral (recommended especially when the ramus profundus is also paralysed)

4. Finally, peroneal nerve paralysis can also be treated with *orthopedic shoes*.

In its least extreme form this could be an orthopedic laced ankle boot with a simple raised heel, an elasticated strip worked into the upper and the back part of the top line (back seam) tilting forward. This shoe is suitable for mild paralysis only; its main advantage is its unobtrusiveness.

The *high peroneal boot* is at the other end of the scale in certain respects. Not only is it very obtrusive, but it is also suitable for severe paralysis and is extremely robust. It comprises an 18 cm (7.2 inch) upper, a paralysis heel counter made of moulded leather with recesses for the malleoli so as not to impair ankle movement, a round-edge heel (buffer heel) and a metatarsal bar incorporated in the compensatory support (Fig. 58). Major disadvantages of this shoe are its extreme weight and its minimal visual appeal, factors which virtually exclude its use in female patients.

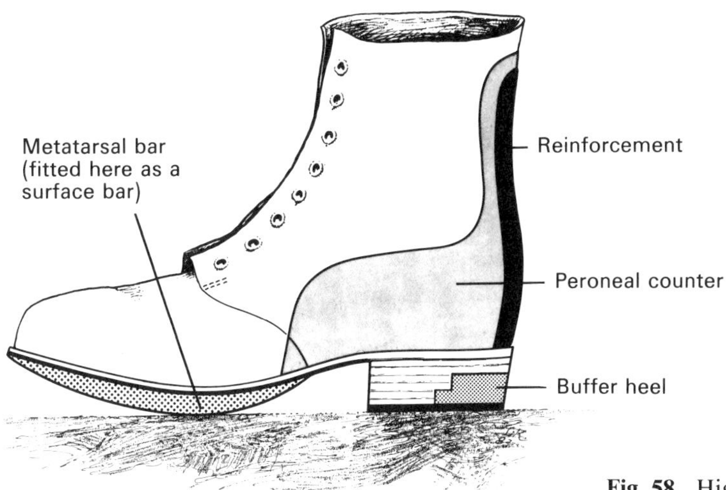

Fig. 58. High peroneal boot

The Kraus peroneal boot is a modification of the high peroneal boot. In this case the upper is only 12 cm (4.8 inches) high, the paralysis counter is lower and the top line of the upper tapers down as it extends forward. This shoe also has a metatarsal bar built into the compensatory support and a round-edge heel (buffer heel). It is more lightweight than the high peroneal boot and can be dorsiflexed more easily but is less robust. Even severe paralysis can be efficiently controlled with this boot.

The orthopedic low shoe with a leather-covered Heidelberg angle and the Vienna shoe have fallen into virtual disuse today because they have been superseded by the other corrective measures described above. The Heidelberg angle is a steel strip which extends from the sole of the foot round the back of the heel and ends just short of the top line of the shoe. It is the oldest method employed in the management of peroneal nerve paralysis and has been in use since the First World War. The shoe accommodating the Heidelberg angle should also have a round-edge heel and a metatarsal bar. It has minimal cosmetic appeal.

The Vienna shoe is a laced ankle boot with an elasticated strip under the lacing; this strip is attached to a strap which is located at the top line of the upper and passes round the lower leg. This shoe should also have a metatarsal bar and round-edge heel as orthopedic elements.

The prescription in peroneal nerve paralysis must take account of the medical aspects (e.g. the degree of paralysis), cosmetic appeal and the need for any special robustness. The following prescription recommendations do not take all these considerations into account:

The Breidbach bandage is recommended in *mild foot-drop* because it is cosmetically unobtrusive.

Rx: One Breidbach internal shoe left (with profiled footplate, peroneal spring, and elasticated strips to raise the tip of the foot).
Diagnosis: Mild peroneal nerve paralysis left.

The simple orthopedic laced ankle boot is also relatively unobtrusive.

Rx: One pair of made-to-measure orthopedic laced ankle boots, with elasticated strip worked into the left upper and with the back seam inclining slightly forward.
Diagnosis: Mild peroneal nerve paralysis left.

The Breidbach bandage may also be used in *moderately severe foot-drop* where cosmetic appeal is a special priority. However, any cosmetic advantage is offset by a slight functional deficit. The same applies with the simple orthopedic laced ankle boot.

The Kraus internal shoe permits a certain degree of compromise between cosmetic appeal and function in such cases.

Rx: One Kraus internal shoe for the left foot (with leather upper, laced closure with elastic strip, and plantar flexion in the ankle joint counteracted by an elastic angled stiffener which extends from under the sole of the foot round the back of the heel and up past the malleoli, bifurcating in the calcaneal region. Profile-moulded footplate.) In addition, one pair of made-to-measure orthopedic shoes with metatarsal bars right and left and buffer heels.
Diagnosis: Moderately severe foot-drop left.

In functional terms, toe-raising springs are especially effective in moderately severe peroneal nerve paralysis, although they are rather more obtrusive than the Breidbach bandage.

Rx: One toe-raising spring left, made of plastic from a plaster cast (where appropriate, with a surface metatarsal bar as a modification to the retail shoe and a slightly raised buffer heel).
Diagnosis: Moderately severe foot-drop.

Where the deep peroneal nerve is also paralysed, the Lehneis spiral is recommended:

Rx: One Lehneis spiral (casting resin) for the left leg, encasing the lateral part of the left heel like a stirrup and spiralling upwards behind the calf.
Diagnosis: Peroneal nerve paralysis left (with involvement of the deep peroneal nerve).

The prescription of a Kraus peroneal boot is justified even in moderately severe paralysis.

Rx: One pair of orthopedic shoes, made to measure, with the left one fashioned as a Kraus peroneal boot (12 cm/4.8 inch upper, moulded leather stabilising heel counter, shock-absorbent heel and compensatory support incorporating metatarsal bar).
Diagnosis: Peroneal nerve paralysis left.

The Breidbach bandage and the Kraus internal shoe may even be used in *severe peroneal nerve paralysis* for patients for whom cosmetic appearance is considered more important than function. The same of course applies with toe-raising springs. However, patients who work outdoors should be supplied with a high peroneal boot.

Rx: One pair of orthopedic shoes, plaster cast, with 18 cm/7.2 inch upper and a paralysis counter extending to just below the top line of the upper, with buffer heel and compensatory support with incorporated metatarsal bar. Shoe bottom with slight outside flare.
Diagnosis: Total peroneal nerve paralysis.

The shoe can be made to exert a pronating effect by displacing the shoe bottom (laterally at an angle) or by stiffening the shoe bottom beyond the metatarsophalangeal joints of the fourth and fifth toes. These modifications are indicated where there is an increased tendency for the foot to supinate as a result of the loss of deep peroneal nerve function.

5.5.2 Tibial and Peroneal Nerve Paralysis

Where all the muscles acting on the foot are paralysed, the *Rabl rigid rocker-sole shoe* (see Fig. 46) is probably the only means of restoring a relatively satisfactory gait pattern.

5.5.3 Femoral Nerve Paralysis

In footwear terms, the simplest method of correcting femoral nerve paralysis is to fit a *toe bar* as a modification to the retail shoe. Because the toe bar bends the sole of the foot upwards, a stiffened shoe bottom beyond the metatarsophalangeal joints should also be prescribed together with a supination wedge. Sometimes the locking effect of the shoe bottom which has been stiffened well forward is sufficient on its own.

When genu recurvatum is present, a raised heel is of prime importance. Its height should be adjusted to suit the individual circumstances (see 5.4.4).

5.5.4 Tibial Nerve Paralysis

This has been dealt with under 5.1.3.2 in connection with pes calcaneoexcavatus due to paralysis.

5.6 Care of the Foot Amputation Stump

Loss of the great toe or of part of the foot in the metatarsal or tarsal region is characterised in functional mechanical terms by shortening of the anterior lever arm, and this is more important than might appear initially. Not only does the anterior foot lever need to be of normal length to produce a normal gait, but the care of foot amputation stumps depends on their capacity to bear weight or stress. This in turn is closely related to scar location and the position of the stump vis-à-vis the lower leg. The orthopedic management of an equinus clubfoot position, for example, is highly complicated: the same applies in stumps with tender scars in the region of the anterior border of the sole.

In principle, foot amputation stumps can be managed with an orthopedic shoe, an internal shoe prosthesis or a forefoot prosthesis.

It was mentioned earlier that metatarsal stumps are most efficiently managed with an orthopedic shoe whereas tarsal stumps require an internal shoe. However, this can only ever be a rough guide because differences in stump length are not the only major criterion. Cosmetic considerations, for example, or the patient's occupation are similarly important. Nevertheless, the following *general guidelines* may be given:

1. In principle, the anterior lever arm can be substituted either by a stiffened full-length sole or by an elastic forefoot filler. In the former case an adequately high metatarsal bar guarantees proper rollover, and in the latter case this function is fulfilled by a sole stiffener which extends from the rear of the foot to just behind the theoretical joint line and whose leading edge then angles sharply up towards the dorsum of the foot (see Fig. 62). Rollover then occurs at this leading edge which is at right angles to the longitudinal axis of the foot.

2. All dead movement between the stump and the orthopedic elements must be eliminated – a particularly difficult task with foot stumps. The following measures may be used to eliminate dead movement:
   a) Support the heel in calcaneus.
   b) Press the stump against the heel counter by using strapping or internal fastening systems.
   c) Employ a heel counter which grips the heel firmly.
   d) Place cushioning material only in the region of the anterior rounded end of the stump but not underneath the stump itself.

3. The shorter the stump, the greater the need for the heel to be supported in calcaneus because the tendency for the stump to plantar flex increases with the extent of foot loss. Similarly, active plantar flexion is only rendered possible by placing the hindfoot in calcaneus.

4. The shorter the stump, the longer the force transmission plate extending from the foot prosthesis to the lower leg (this principle is most clearly illustrated in the Teufel forefoot prosthesis, see 5.6.2.6).

5. The stump can only be supported accurately by preparing a plaster-cast impression.

5.6.1 Management of Individual Types of Foot Stump

It will be helpful first to review the means available for the management of different anatomical types of stump and then to discuss the various types of management in detail. In terms of anatomical and functional mechanics, there are five categories of toe or foot loss (long and short metatarsal stumps and long and short tarsal stumps will be counted as two categories instead of four).

1. *Loss of a great toe* can be compensated by a modification to the retail shoe in conjunction with an insert. The prescription is simple.

Rx: One pair of made-to-measure aluminium inserts with a hallux flange extending forward to the toe end of the left shoe and resilient, cushioned hallux prosthesis left.
Diagnosis: Loss of left hallux.

2. Where *all the toes have been lost,* a low orthopedic shoe is indicated.

3. The care of *long and short metatarsal stumps* is rather more complicated. The following possibilities may be considered:
   a) *The simple shoe for foot amputees.* This is relatively lightweight (Fig. 59) but has the disadvantage of containing only few orthopedic elements

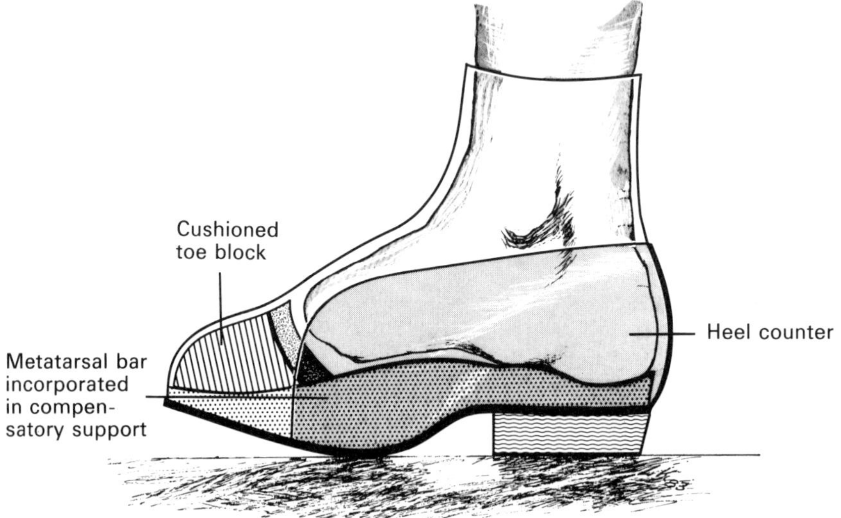

Fig. 59. Simple shoe for foot amputees

which can exert any major influence on gait. It is thus in fact a leisure shoe which also has reasonable cosmetic appeal.

b) *The classical foot amputation shoe* (Fig. 60) is designed as a working shoe. It is robust and hardly limits ankle joint mobility at all, but is relatively heavy and does not guarantee an absolutely smooth gait pattern.

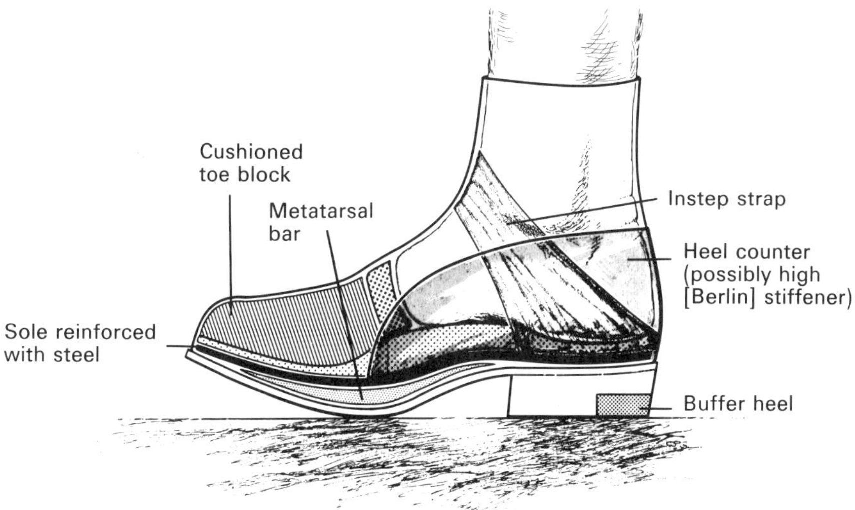

Fig. 60. Classical foot amputation shoe

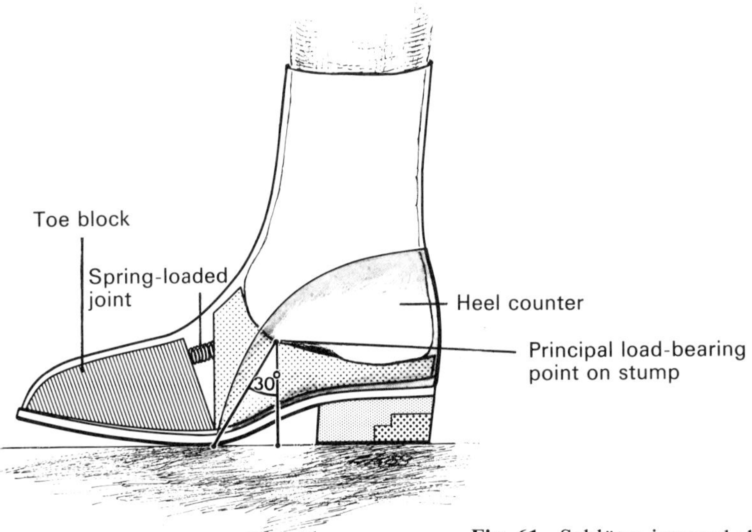

Fig. 61. Schlüter internal shoe prosthesis

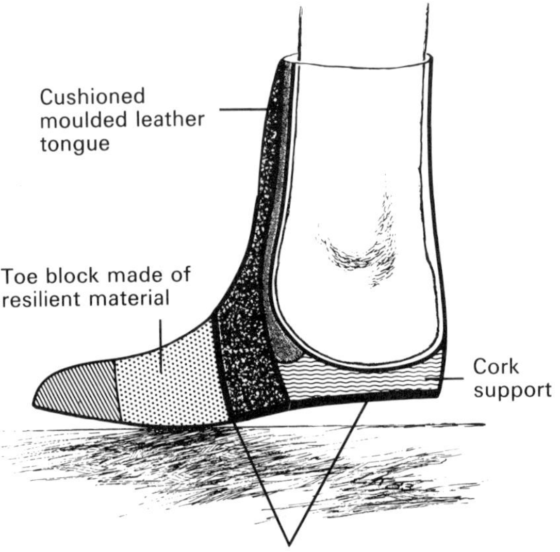

Fig. 62. Welsch internal shoe prosthesis

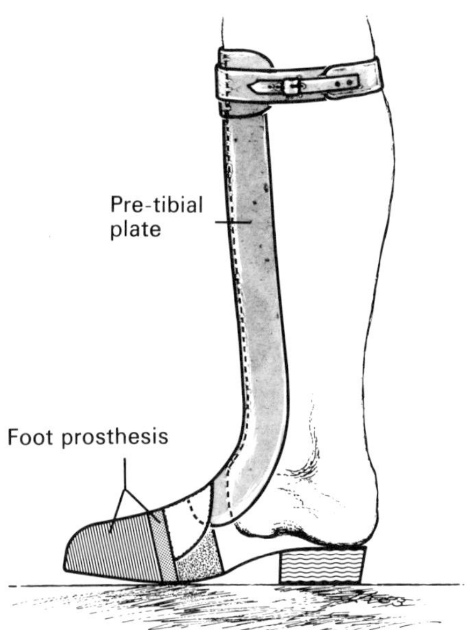

Fig. 63. Teufel internal shoe prosthesis

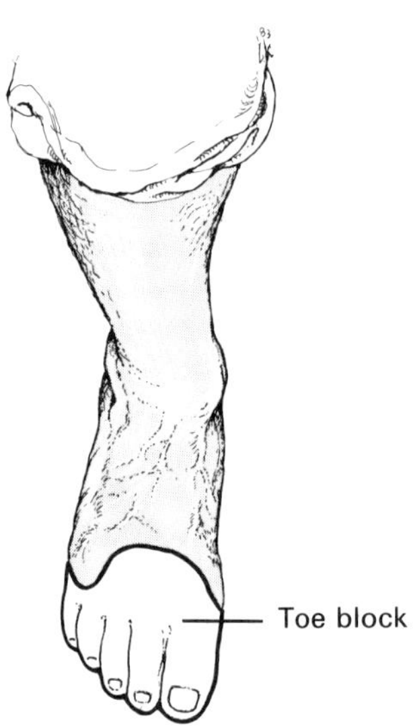

Fig. 64. Use of a toe block to replace missing toes

c) *The Schlüter internal shoe prosthesis* (Fig. 61) is very light and also satisfies cosmetic requirements. The patient is able to wear retail shoes. However, because it is not particularly robust, it is not really suitable for heavy physical work.

d) *The Welsch internal shoe prosthesis* (Fig. 62) satisfies functional and cosmetic requirements equally well. It is more robust than the Schlüter internal shoe, but is heavier and necessitates orthopedic custom-made shoes.

e) In theory, long or short metatarsal stumps could be catered for using a *Teufel internal shoe prosthesis* (Fig. 63). As a rule, however, this should be reserved for long and short tarsal stumps and for Pirogoff amputations.

4. *Long and short tarsal stumps* can also be accommodated using:
a) *The simple shoe for foot amputees* in cases where the gait pattern does not need correction and where functional substitution by orthopedic elements is unnecessary.

b) *The Schlüter internal shoe prosthesis* should be used for long tarsal stumps only, not for short ones.

c) *The Welsch internal shoe prosthesis* is also suitable for short stumps.

d) *The Teufel forefoot prosthesis* (Fig. 63) is the most robust of all prostheses but is not ideal for use in female patients because it is too obtrusive. It should be prescribed together with an orthopedic, custom-made shoe (laced ankle boot).

e) If designed as a working shoe, the *Rabl rigid rocker-sole shoe* (see Fig. 46) may occasionally be considered for *short tarsal stumps*. This shoe is particularly robust but does immobilise the ankle joint completely; it does not permit a smooth, non-limping gait.

5. The *Pirogoff stump* can be accommodated using a *Welsch* or *Teufel* internal shoe prosthesis or a *Rabl rigid rocker-sole shoe*. The advantages and limitations listed above also apply here. The *Teufel* forefoot prosthesis is particularly well suited for this type of stump because it yields the best functional results.

5.6.2 Footwear for Amputation Stumps

5.6.2.1 Orthopedic Shoe for Loss of All Toes

As in loss of the hallux, metatarsophalangeal joint function is disturbed, the difference being that toe-off is even more impaired. A *toe filler* (Fig. 64), an *orthopedic bar* and a *stiffened sole* are the major compensatory elements and these can be accommodated most effectively in an orthopedic shoe.

Rx: One pair of made-to measure low orthopedic shoes with compensatory support left, incorporating a metatarsal pad, support in front of the calcaneus and a cushioned toe filler; with a rocker bar positioned proximal to the end of the stump and a reinforced sole. Metatarsal bar right.
Diagnosis: Loss of all toes on left foot.

5.6.2.2 Simple Shoe for Partial Foot Amputees

The only orthopedic elements in this shoe are a cushioned toe block, a metatarsal bar and support in front of the calcaneus (see Fig. 59).

Rx: One pair of orthopedic shoes with compensatory support, with special support in front of the calcaneus, an orthopedic bar and a cushioned toe block. Reinforced toe cap and heel counter. Metatarsal bar right.
Diagnosis: Loss of left foot in metatarsal region.

5.6.2.3 Classical Foot Amputation Shoe

Internal fastening is required here because of the increased likelihood of dead movement inside the shoe. The shorter the stump, the higher the ideal upper (at least 18 cm/7.2 inches). The heel counter may be reinforced as a paralysis counter and the foot stump should be supported in calcaneus. The outsole should be of the non-slip variety because its contact surface with the ground is reduced. The reinforced sole extends from the toe end of the shoe to beyond the waist, which in turn means that the toe spring should be at least 2.5 cm (1 inch). Elastic reinforcement of the tongue is indicated in short metatarsal stumps (see Fig. 60).

Rx: One pair of orthopedic shoes (plaster cast) fashioned as a classical foot amputation shoe left (with internal fastening, upper 20 cm (8 inches) high and reinforced with a paralysis counter; sole and waist reinforced with steel; with compensatory support incorporating a metatarsal bar and a foot prosthesis; with a non-slip sole, buffer heel and toe spring at least 2.5 cm (1 inch) high). Metatarsal bar right.
Diagnosis: Left foot amputated in the metatarsal region.

5.6.2.4 Schlüter Internal Shoe Prosthesis

This type of orthopedic appliance features a wooden foot prosthesis, the two sections of which are linked by a spring-loaded joint. It is designed in such a way that, during the swing phase of ambulation, the distal section plantar flexes at a transverse joint on the sole of the prosthesis, thus creating a dorsal, V-shaped segment. This segment disappears again during rollover following passive impact of the two wooden sections and thus limits the extent of dorsiflexion. The V-shaped segment is located anterior to the tip of the stump. The position of the rotational axis is determined by subtending an angle of 30° from an anterior load-bearing point on the stump tip. One arm of this angle represents the perpendicular from the load-bearing point to the ground. The point at which the other arm intersects the shoe bottom represents the apex of the V-shape and hence its rotational axis (see Fig. 61).

The prosthesis is combined with a laced upper and a heel counter which encase the foot and hold it in calcaneus. The prosthesis is also known as an *Orfi prosthesis*. The prescription is straightforward:

Rx: One Schlüter internal shoe prosthesis left (Orfi prosthesis).
Diagnosis: Left foot amputated in the metatarsal region.

5.6.2.5 Welsch Internal Shoe Prosthesis

The major elements here are:

1. A foot prosthesis made of a robust, resilient material.

2. Compensatory support to hold the foot in calcaneus.

3. A metal plate which extends forward under the compensatory support and then bends dorsally at right angles, passing in front of the stump and into the resilient foot prosthesis. Push-off occurs where the plate bends at right angles; if this point is located approximately 2 cm (0.8 inches) behind the metatarsophalangeal joints (measured on the healthy foot), an almost normal foot lever action is achieved. However, this cannot always be guaranteed.

4. The *Welsch* internal shoe prosthesis also has a tongue of varying stiffness and height which transmits bodyweight partially on to the foot prosthesis.

5. An internal shoe encases the stump itself (see Fig. 62).

Rx: One pair of made-to-measure orthopedic shoes and a Welsch internal shoe prosthesis left.
Diagnosis: Short tarsal stump left.

5.6.2.6 Teufel Forefoot Prosthesis

The prime feature of this prosthesis is that it bears the load during rollover whereas the stump takes over the bodyweight during stance and heel-strike. The prosthesis comprises the following elements:

1. A foot prosthesis, the tip of which is made of a resilient material.

2. A supportive plate which sits loosely against the anterior aspect of the lower leg and is attached to it proximally by a calf band. This supportive plate (made of metal or casting resin) is loosely connected to the foot prosthesis and extends upwards as far as the head of the tibia. During rollover, it transmits the bodyweight load loosely to the prosthesis.

3. Where appropriate, an internal upper may be required to bring about a closer union between the prosthesis and the stump. Frequently, however, the orthopedic shoe alone is able to fulfil this function (see Fig. 63).

Rx: One pair of made-to-measure orthopedic shoes with a Teufel forefoot prosthesis for the left leg and compensation for the leg length discrepancy.
Diagnosis: Pirogoff amputation left.

The *Rabl* rigid rocker-sole shoe is described in section 5.3.1.

5.7 Shoes for Special Purposes

5.7.1 Shoe Provision for the Lower-Limb Amputee

In contrast to the healthy foot, the joint line of the prosthetic foot does not run obliquely from posterolateral to anteromedial, but is at right angles to the direction of travel. In certain cases, the prescription of an orthopedic shoe for the artificial leg may be justified if the gait pattern cannot be influenced in any other way. Generally, however, the retail shoe is sufficient provided it is modified to improve its functional mechanics, i.e. with a low rocker bar placed slightly further back than usual and at right angles to the direction of travel.

The healthy foot of the lower-limb amputee does not require an orthopedic shoe of its own. However, timely prescription of corrective orthopedic elements as appropriate is essential here too: e.g. an insert with a metatarsal pad for splayfoot, or an insert for planovalgus/planotransversus foot.

5.7.2 Appliance Shoe

Cooperation between the orthopedic shoemaker and the orthopedic technician is essential whenever a leg brace has to be supplied together with an orthopedic shoe. Very frequently (and nowadays more so than in the past) the appliance is preferred to the orthopedic shoe for the compensation of more pronounced leg inequality. In such circumstances, the orthopedic technician corrects the leg inequality with the appliance while the orthopedic shoemaker creates the conditions for rollover on the shoe. Normally, the connecting piece between the leg brace and the shoe is a shoe plate which is incorporated between the heel and the insole. The shoe plate then generally has a simple snap-in joint at the ankle which articulates with the braces of the appliance. Its rotational axis lies directly in front of the tip of the lateral malleolus. The appliance shoe should generally have good rollover properties which can also be exploited to compensate for leg length inequality. If the ankle joint is immobilised, a round-edge heel and a metatarsal bar are needed, as for a rocker-sole shoe.

Similar features are appropriate for all other types of leg appliance. Prescription generally presents no difficulties and can invariably be kept brief: however, explicit reference to the type of orthopedic bars required in each case is a minimum requirement.

5.7.3 Bath Shoe

In certain foot deformities the patient is able to walk barefoot only with extreme difficulty or severe discomfort. The bath shoe is indicated here to permit walking on the beach or at the swimming baths, and especially to facilitate free participation in therapeutic water exercises.

The bath shoe may incorporate all the orthopedic elements which an orthopedic town shoe might have. It is manufactured from watertight plastic material and should have an especially snug fit. The upper is usually made of a softish, rubber-like substance.

The prescription should be based on the existing last. However, two things should be remembered. Firstly, the allowances on the last (such as are almost always necessary for orthopedic town shoes) should be less pronounced than usual. Secondly, a casting resin last rather than a wooden last is generally required for a bath shoe. A second last may therefore have to be made.

6 Approval of the Orthopedic Shoe by the Physician

The acceptability of the orthopedic shoe should be tested by reconsidering all those points which formed the basis for its prescription. In other words, the impediment should be related in some measure to its potential for compensation with orthopedic elements, and the physician should verify that these are adequate and have been fitted properly. It is therefore recommended that a fitting session be arranged together with the orthopedic shoemaker while the shoe is still being made so that any errors emerging can be corrected at an early stage and so that the prescribed orthopedic elements can be tested for function. The patient's comfort should also naturally be taken into account and the perpendicular construction of the shoe should be checked. These same questions should be asked again during final inspection of the finished shoe. It is advisable to work through a specific checklist.

1. It is best to begin by forming an approximate, but generally indicative impression of the *patient's gait*. Attention should be paid to the following points:
   a) Does rollover match up to expectations and, where appropriate, has it been corrected? Does the patient limp?
   b) Is the angle of foot placement correct? Normally, the foot is rotated outwards by about $10°$ from the direction of travel.
   c) Is stride length consistent with the residual function of the leg?
   d) Is heel-strike essentially normal?
   e) How does the toe-off phase look?
   f) How does the patient feel in his new shoes? Does he complain of localised pressure, and does he also feel that his gait is easier? Does he now find it easier to stand?

2. Care should next be taken to ensure that the prescribed *orthopedic elements* have also been incorporated correctly and that each fulfils its respective mechanical function.

3. *Shoe length* must be checked. It is a common error for shoes to turn out too short because insufficient allowance has been made on the last. In this context, reliance should not be placed entirely on the subjective comments of the patient. Objective verification should also be made to ensure that the toes are not pinched against the end of the shoe and that no excessive pressure is exerted at the heel. *Shoe width* must also be checked, not forgetting that the compensatory support is in position.

4. The *compensatory support* should then be removed and positioned against the foot to ensure that it fits well.

5. The *height of the upper* should be inspected because it is not uncommon (particularly if not specified in the prescription) for this to be made higher than is absolutely necessary. In peroneal nerve paralysis, however, there is a certain minimum height, and in foot amputation this can be as much as 18 cm (7.2 inches), measured over the medial malleolus.

6. Is the *heel height* consistent with the *toe spring?*

7. Have the *principles of perpendicular shoe construction* been followed?

It is no simple matter if the gait pattern or the patient's comments indicate unmistakably that the shoe falls short of expectations. In such circumstances it is not always easy to detect the error at the first attempt or, conversely, to decide whether the patient might not be anticipating too much. Certain shortcomings, e.g. areas of localised pressure, are relatively simple to rectify. The situation generally becomes most complex in cases where the shoe is designed to facilitate or correct the function of several muscle groups or joints, for example, in flaccid paralysis, always assuming that an (additional) orthopedic appliance might not be more appropriate in the first place. There should then be fresh consideration as to whether the individual orthopedic elements are genuinely sufficient to compensate for the functional deficit or whether they might not be mutually counterproductive. Renewed consultation with the shoemaker may also be necessary to discuss the correct perpendicular and functional construction of the shoe.

7 Correction Principles –
A Review

The principal indications for the individual orthopedic elements will be reviewed briefly in this final short chapter. Less emphasis has been placed here on completeness than on the frequency, and hence the importance, of the respective modifications and disorders.

It is hoped that these pages will enable the reader to review simply and conveniently the individual orthopedic shoe possibilities for specific disorders.

Hip Joint

1. *Shortening stride length:* Raised heels
2. *Reducing jarring:* Buffer heels

Extending the Knee (in Quadriceps Weakness)

1. Toe bar
2. Totally stiffened shoe bottom
3. Flat heels
4. Stiffened tongue
5. Tibial plate

Flexing the Knee

1. Raised heels
2. Buffer heels
3. Metatarsal bar moved back slightly

Compensation for Stiffened Knee Joint

1. Lengthen healthy leg by 2 cm (0.8 inches)
2. Metatarsal bar on affected leg
3. Soft buffer heels

4. Rocker-sole shoe with centre of rocker sole arc located at the midpoint
   of the hip joint

Relief of Genu Valgum

1. Medial heel flare
2. Supination wedge
3. Snugly fitting upper

Relief of Genu Varum

Caution essential in cases with concurrent planovalgus feet! Therefore, with
qualification:
Lateral heel flare

Stimulation of Calf Muscles

Flat heels

Sparing Calf Muscles (e.g. in peripheral vascular disease)

Raised heels

Compensation for Leg Inequality

1. Thicker outsole and raised heel
2. Orthopedic shoe
3. Internal shoe
4. O'Connor boot

Limiting Movement in Ankle Joint

1. Raised heels
2. Metatarsal bar
3. Round-edge heel
4. Round-ankle stiffener
5. Rigid rocker-sole shoe

Compensation for Reduced Movement in Ankle Joint

1. Metatarsal bar
2. Round-edge heel
3. Rocker-sole shoe

Facilitating Plantar Flexion

1. Behind-heel float
2. Metatarsal bar moved back slightly
3. Raised heels

Limiting Plantar Flexion

Peroneal counter (see under peroneal nerve paralysis)

Limiting Dorsiflexion of the Foot

Stiffened tongue

Facilitating Dorsiflexion of the Foot

Buffer heel

Relieving Pressure on the Calcaneus

1. Raised heels
2. Buffer heel

Preventing Hindfoot Collapse

1. Flared heel
2. Flared sole and heel
3. Snugly fitting heel counter
4. Laterally or medially displaced heel

Supinating Effect on the Foot

1. Sole displaced medially (at an angle)
2. Medial sole stiffener
3. Supination wedge has a supinating effect on the hindfoot and a pronating effect on the forefoot
4. Medial sole wedging

Pronating Effect on the Foot

1. Sole displaced laterally (at an angle)
2. Lateral sole stiffener beyond the metatarsophalangeal joint of the fourth and fifth toes
3. Lateral sole wedging

Discouraging Supination

Heel and sole displaced laterally

Discouraging Pronation

Heel and sole displaced medially

Inward or Outward Rotation of the Foot

1. Triangular bar
2. Lateral sole stiffener has an inward-rotating and pronating action
3. Medial sole stiffener has an outward-rotating and supinating action

Immobilisation (Pressure Relief) in Tarsal Joints

1. Cradle-shaped wedge heel
2. Metatarsal bar moved back slightly (inhibits painful bending during final stage of rollover)
3. Heel raise (reduces pronatory and supinatory movement)
4. Support under sustentaculum tali
5. Stiffened sole (reduces transmission of effects of uneven terrain and has an immobilising action)
6. Flared heel (counteracts tilting)
7. Buffer heel (absorbs energy on impact)
8. Stable and snug heel counter (reduces calcaneal tilting)
9. Upper which encases the metatarsus softly but firmly (prevents movement inside shoe)
10. Rocker-sole shoe

Extension of Hammer Toes

1. Metatarsal pad
2. Felt ring pads

Compensation for Impaired Metatarsophalangeal Joint Mobility

Rocker sole

Limiting Metatarsophalangeal Joint Mobility

1. Stiffened sole
2. Rocker bar

Correcting Splayfoot

Metatarsal pad

Relief of Pressure in Splayfoot

Horseshoe bar

Relief of Pressure on Sesamoid Bone

L-shaped bar

Modifications in Relatively Severe Foot Deformity

1. Stepped insole
2. Moulded insole
3. Internal shoe
4. Special attention to perpendicular construction

Increasing Sole Contact Surface

Moulded insole

Reducing Sole Contact Surface

Stepped insole

Preventing the Foot from Slipping Inside Shoe

1. Internal fastening or Eisenmann strap
2. Roughened whole-length sock

3. Upper which firmly encases the metatarsal region
4. Toe grip bar (especially in equinus)
5. Support in front of the calcaneus

Stabilising the Waist of the Shoe

1. Wedge heel
2. Stiffened sole
3. Heel with central waist support
4. Thomas heel

Increasing the Ground Contact Surface of Shoe

1. Wedge heel
2. Heel with central waist support
3. Flared heel

Mechanical Toe Protection

Stiffened toe cap

Transfer of Gravitational Force to Shoe

Stiffened tongue

Transfer of Gravitational Force to Foot Prosthesis

Anterior tibial plate

Facilitating Rollover

1. Round-edge heel (buffer heel)
2. Cradle-shaped wedge heel
3. Metatarsal bar
4. Rocker bar

(Fore)Foot Prostheses

See 5.6.

Glossary

Adduction	Movement of the foot toward the central axis of the body.
Ankylosis	Total stiffening or fixation of a joint due to pathological processes (see Arthrodesis).
Arthrodesis	Total stiffening or fixation of a joint by operative means.
Arthrosis	A degenerative process in a joint, accompanied by cartilage destruction.
Ataxia	A loss of the ability to perform smooth and coordinated movements, characterised by incoordination in the muscles of the extremities due to a neurological lesion.
Chopart's joint	Joint between the talus and calcaneus posteriorly and the navicular and cuboid bones anteriorly (S-shaped).
Contracture	Restriction of movement in a joint. Used in combination with another descriptor to indicate the position where mobility is limited, e.g. flexion contracture = inability to flex (completely).
Destruction, mutilating	Mutilating deformity of the toes (due to chronic rheumatoid arthritis).
Detorsion	A condition in which the foot is rotated laterally out of physiological torsion.
Dorsal	Relating to or toward the upper surface or back of the foot.
Dorsiflexion	Raising the toes and forepart of the foot, by extension at the ankle joint (= dorsal extension).
Elephantiasis	Pronounced enlargement of a part of the body, usually the result of lymphatic obstruction.
Femoral nerve paralysis	Paralysis of the femoral nerve in which normal extension of the lower leg at the knee is no longer possible (see N. femoralis).

Fibular deviation	Lateral deviation of the metatarsophalangeal joints (due to chronic rheumatoid arthritis).
Flange	An elevated piece at the medial or lateral edge of a shoe insert.
Frontal	In a direction parallel to the forehead and dividing the body into anterior and posterior portions, i. e. at right angles to a sagittal (q. v.) plane.
Genu recurvatum	A condition of hyperextension of the knee.
Hallux rigidus	Painful restriction of the range of movement in the first metatarsophalangeal joint, frequently secondary to degenerative joint changes.
Hallux valgus	A deformity of the great toe in which the first metatarsophalangeal joint deviates toward the lateral border of the foot.
Indication	A symptom or circumstance that indicates the advisability or necessity of a particular procedure or treatment.
Lateral	Relating to or toward the outer border of the foot.
Metatarsal	Relating to the metatarsus or forepart of the foot.
Metatarsal head	Head of a metatarsal bone. The expanded distal end of a metatarsal bone that articulates with the proximal phalanx of the same digit.
Medial	Relating to or toward the inner border of the foot.
M. quadriceps	See Quadriceps.
N. femoralis	Femoral nerve. Supplies the quadriceps muscle of the thigh (see Quadriceps).
N. peroneus	Peroneal nerve, with a deep (ramus profundus) and a superficial (ramus superficialis) branch. The deep branch raises the foot and toes, and the superficial branch raises the lateral border of the foot (see Peroneal nerve paralysis).
Orthotic	An orthopedic appliance, e. g. brace appliance for a leg.
Paralysis, flaccid	Muscle paralysis due to injury to nerve supply, accompanied by loss of muscle tone, e. g. femoral nerve paralysis (q. v.).
Paralysis, spastic	See Spasticity.
Paresis	(Partial or incomplete) paralysis.
Patella	Kneecap.

Peroneal nerve paralysis	Paralysis of the nerves of the lower leg, as a result of which dorsiflexion of the foot is no longer possible (see N. peroneus and Dorsiflexion).
Pes adductus	A deformity of the foot in which the forepart of the foot is angled away from the main longitudinal axis of the foot toward the midline.
Pes calcaneoexcavatus	A calcaneus deformity of the foot in which there is also a cavus component.
Pes cavus	A deformity of the foot characterised by an abnormally high longitudinal arch.
Pes equinoexcavatus	A deformity of the foot characterised by fixed plantar flexion and a high longitudinal arch.
Pes equinus	Permanent plantar flexion of the foot so that the weight of the body rests on the anterior portion of the foot only.
Pes planotransversus	A deformity of the foot characterised by flattening of the longitudinal and transverse arches.
Pes planovalgus	A deformity of the foot characterised by flattening of the longitudinal arch and eversion.
Pirogoff amputation	Amputation of the foot, the lower articular surfaces of the tibia and fibula being sawn through and the ends covered with a portion of the calcaneus which has also been sawn through from above posteriorly downward and forward.
Plantar	Relating to or toward the sole of the foot.
Plantar aponeurosis	A tendinous sheet extending along the sole of the foot from the calcaneus to the metatarsal heads.
Plantar flexion	Downward movement of the foot and ankle, i.e. toward the sole of the foot.
Pretibial	Relating to the anterior portion of the lower leg (shin bone).
Pronation	Eversion of the sole of the foot so that the lateral border is elevated and the medial border is lowered.
Quadriceps	Quadriceps muscle of the anterior region of the thigh; extends the lower leg (see Femoral nerve paralysis).
Ray	The phalanges of a toe, together with the corresponding metatarsal (and tarsal) bones.
Resultant	An effective force that results from the cooperation and antagonism of varied individual forces.

Sagittal	In an anteroposterior (or posteroanterior) direction, i.e. at right angles to the frontal plane.
Spasticity	A state of exaggerated spasmodic (involuntary) muscle tone due to a disturbance in the neurological pathways of the brain and spinal cord. Spasticity may follow a stroke or be a congenital condition.
Supination	Inversion of the sole of the foot so that the lateral border is lowered and the medial border is elevated.
Sustentaculum tali	A bracket-like lateral bony projection from the medial surface of the calcaneus.
Talipes calcaneus	Permanent dorsiflexion of the foot so that the weight of the body rests on the heel only.
Talocrural joint	Ankle joint.
Tibial nerve paralysis	Paralysis of the tibial nerves, characterised by a functional deficit of the muscles of the calf and sole of the foot. The foot is permanently dorsiflexed and cannot undergo plantar flexion. Underlying cause of talipes calcaneus.
Torsion	(Normal) rotation of the forefoot in pronation and of the hindfoot in supination.
Trochanter, greater	Bony prominence at the upper and lateral part of the shaft of the femur. Can usually be palpated beneath the skin.
Valgus	A position in which a limb or joint is turned outward to an abnormal degree, resulting in lateral concavity.
Varus	A position in which a limb or joint is turned inward to an abnormal degree, resulting in medial concavity.
Wedging, lateral	Raising the lateral rim of the shoe bottom.
Wedging, medial	Raising the medial rim of the shoe bottom.

Bibliography

Baumgartner R (1972) Die orthopädietechnische Versorgung des Fußes. Thieme, Stuttgart

Hegenauer H (1981) Fachkunde für lederverarbeitende Berufe (5th edition). Heyer, Essen

Henkel F (1979) Zurichtung des Konfektionsschuhes. In: Imhäuser G (ed) Der Fuß. Vordruckverlag, Bruchsal, p 425

Hohmann D, Uhlig R (1982) Orthopädische Technik (7th edition). Enke, Stuttgart

Kraus E (1973) Biomechanik und Schuhtechnik. Maurer, Geislingen

Kraus E (1980) Fachkunde Orthopädieschuhtechnik (3rd edition). Maurer, Geislingen

Lange M, Hipp E (1976) Lehrbuch der Orthopädie und Traumatologie. Enke, Stuttgart

Marquardt W (1965) Die theoretischen Grundlagen der Orthopädie-Schuhmacherei (2nd edition). Maurer, Geislingen

Marquardt W (1981) Orthopädische Schuhe und Schuheinlagen. In: Witt A, Rettig H, Schlegel KF, Hackenbroch M, Hupfauer W (eds) Orthopädie in Praxis und Klinik (vol 2/19). Thieme, Stuttgart New York, p 1

Meyer E (1974) Moderne Arbeitstechniken im Orthopädieschuhmacherhandwerk. Maurer, Geislingen

Münzenberg KJ (1981) Orthopädie in der Praxis, edition medizin, Weinheim

Rabl CRH (1951) Orthopädische Schuhe und Stützeinlagen. Enke, Stuttgart

Rabl CH, Nyga W (1982) Orthopädie des Fußes (6th edition). Enke, Stuttgart

Regenspurger G (1975) Orthopädische Einlagen- und Schuhversorgung. Barth, Leipzig

Thomsen W (1966) Pflege deine Füße – gesunde Füße, gesunder Mensch. Thieme, Stuttgart

Weil S, Weil UH (1966) Mechanik des Gehens. Thieme, Stuttgart

Index